Essentials of Abdomino-Pelvic Sonography

Essentials of Abdomino-Pelvic Sonography

A Handbook for Practitioners

Dr. Swati Goyal

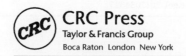

CRC Press
Taylor & Francis Group
Boca Raton London New York

CRC Press is an imprint of the
Taylor & Francis Group, an **informa** business

CRC Press
Taylor & Francis Group
6000 Broken Sound Parkway NW, Suite 300
Boca Raton, FL 33487-2742

First issued in paperback 2020

ISBN-13: 978-0-367-57230-3 (pbk)
ISBN-13: 978-1-138-50182-9 (hbk)

Library of Congress Cataloging-in-Publication Data

Names: Goyal, Swati, author.
Title: Essentials of abdomino-pelvic sonography : a handbook for
practitioners / Dr. Swati Goyal.
Description: Boca Raton, FL : CRC Press/Taylor & Francis Group, [2018] |
Includes bibliographical references and index.
Identifiers: LCCN 2017034325| ISBN 9781138501829 (hardback : alk. paper) |
ISBN 9781351261203 (ebook : alk. paper)
Subjects: | MESH: Digestive System Diseases--diagnostic imaging |
Abdomen--diagnostic imaging | Pelvis--diagnostic imaging | Ultrasonography
| Ultrasonography, Prenatal
Classification: LCC RC78.7.U4 | NLM WI 141 | DDC 617.5/50754--dc23
LC record available at https://lccn.loc.gov/2017034325

Visit the Taylor & Francis Web site at
http://www.taylorandfrancis.com

and the CRC Press Web site at
http://www.crcpress.com

Dedication

Dedicated to my adorable kids, Prisha and Rushank, who invigorated me in spite of all the time the task of book writing took me away from them.

Contents

List of Abbreviations

USG	ultrasonography		RA	right atrium
MHz	megahertz		RV	right ventricle
KHz	kilohertz		LA	left atrium
PE	piezoelectric effect		LV	left ventricle
IVC	inferior vena cava		AFI	amniotic fluid index
GB	gallbladder		AFV	amniotic fluid volume
HCC	hepatocellular carcinoma		IUGR	intrauterine growth retardation
CT	computed tomography		CVS	cardiovascular system
MRI	magnetic resonance imaging		GIT	gastro intestinal system
CBD	common bile duct		CNS	central nervous system
IHBR	intrahepatic biliary radicle		CDUS	color Doppler sonography
RUQ	right upper quadrant		PI	pulsatility index
M:F	male: female		EDV	end diastolic volume
PUJ	pelvi-ureteric junction		PSV	peak systolic velocity
TCC	transitional cell carcinoma		RI	resistive index
RCC	renal cell carcinoma		MCA	middle cerebral artery
UTI	urinary tract infection		ECA	external carotid artery
HRT	hormone replacement therapy		ICA	internal carotid artery
PID	pelvic inflammatory disease		CCA	common carotid artery
OCP	oral contraceptive pills		PV	portal vein
AFP	alpha-fetoprotein		HV	hepatic vein
TAS	transabdominal sonography		SMV	superior mesenteric vein
TVS	transvaginal sonography		SV	splenic vein
LUS	lower uterine segment		H/o	history of
FSH	follicle stimulating hormone		A/w	associated with
LH	luteinizing hormone		D/D	differential diagnosis
GS	gestational sac		C.f.	compare from
MSD	mean sac diameter		S/o	suggestive of
YS	yolk sac		hCG	human chorionic gonadotropin
GA	gestational age		Pap smear	papanikolaou smear
CRL	crown rump length		U/L	unilateral
FHR	fetal heart rate		B/L	bilateral
IVF	in vitro fertilization		EDTA	ethylene diamine tetra acetic acid
BPD	biparietal diameter			
HC	head circumference		ERCP	endoscopic retrograde cholangio pancreatography
AC	abdominal circumference			
FL	femur length		MRCP	magnetic resonance cholangio pancreatography
EFW	effective fetal weight			

CECT	contrast enhanced computed tomography	ACE	angiotensin converting enzyme
CRF	chronic renal failure	pGTN	persistent gestational trophoblastic neoplasia
UPJ	uretero-pelvic junction		
D&C	dilatation & curettage	IUCD	intra-uterine contraceptive device
TOA	tubo-ovarian abscess		
HPV	Human Papilloma Virus	US	ultrasound
DES	Diethylstilbestrol	IVF–ET/GIFT	in vitro fertilization-embryo transfer/gamete intra fallopian transfer
BPH	benign prostatic hyperplasia		
IUP	intrauterine pregnancy		
LVOT	left ventricular outflow tract	FT	fallopian tube
RVOT	right ventricular outflow tract	MDA	mullerian duct anomalies
DWV	dandy walker variant	FB	foreign bodies
UVJ	uretero-vesical junction	NHL	non hodgkin's lymphoma
SVC	superior Venacava	VR	volume rendering

Preface

Sonography has emerged as a substantial milestone in the field of radiodiagnosis, imparting conspicuous contribution to early diagnosis and aiding the management of most of the ailments. The easy availability, noninvasive nature, and cost-effectiveness have led to its necessity as a fundamental tool usually at the first referral level. The number of radiologists and sonologists are not commensurate with that of patients to render proficient technique and interpretation.

Sonography has been recognized as a sine qua non for diagnosis of most of the conditions; hence, its knowledge is desired by the practicing doctors from most of the fields such as medicine, surgery, gynecology, pediatrics, ophthalmology, orthopedics, and so on, apart from radiologists. This book is formulated as a concise teaching guide for general practitioners, sonologists, and resident doctors aspiring for diagnostic medical sonography. Although this book has been drafted mainly for trainee sonologists, the text will be useful to other physicians interested in medical imaging as well.

This book comprises 7 parts and 45 chapters. Part I explains ultrasound physics in an uncomplicated and illustrated manner with basic line diagrams. Part II and III consist of abdominal and obstetric sonography, respectively, and include both normal and abnormal findings with differential diagnosis and relevant images, usually encountered during routine practice, covering each of the body area in different chapters. Parts IV through VI incorporate brief overview of color Doppler, high-resolution sonography, and USG-guided interventions. Doppler findings in obstetrics, carotid vessels, renal artery, portal vein, and peripheral vessels have been described

precisely. High-resolution sonography, including head and neck thyroid, breast, anterior abdominal wall, skin, gastrointestinal system, scrotum, and miscellaneous (ophthalmic and transfontanellar) have been compendiously described. In Part VII, "Recent Advances in Sonography"—3D USG, elastography, tissue harmonic imaging, and transperineal sonography to name a few have been framed, envisaging its future prospects. Succinct account of various routinely experienced pathologies along with suitable images has been enlisted. This book includes sample questions (for competency-based tests [CBT] under pre-conception pre-natal diagnostic techniques [Pc PNDT] in India) and multiple choice questions (MCQs) with an answer key at the end and case reports for practical orientation, on a pattern based on various certificate examinations and CBT for technicians and general practitioners undergoing training for being sonologists.

Being an operator-dependent technique, appropriate training and expertise are required along with the knowledge of sonography. This book is an adjunct to standard textbooks and is not intended to substitute for them.

This book is primarily for residents and doctors pursuing bachelor/masters in medical ultrasound to assist them during their sonography training with a focus on point-wise description of abdomino–pelvic and obstetric imaging and help them in guiding and writing certificate examinations such as American Registry for Diagnostic Medical Sonography (ARDMS) in the United States and Canada, Consortium for Accreditation of Sonographic Evaluation (CASE) accredited ultrasound courses in the United Kingdom, or CBT in India.

Acknowledgments

Albeit I am the sole author, this accomplishment was beyond the bounds of possibility without the support from many individuals who contributed, from images and suggestions to viewpoints, and above all their blessings.

I would thank Dr. R. K. Gupta, MD (Medicine)—an outstanding practitioner and academician, along with a doting father—who taught me the value of education and hard work and inspired me to write this book on sonography for beginners in a language that is easy to comprehend.

Wholehearted appreciation to my husband Dr. Sanjay Goyal, MD (Pediatrics), IAS, and a visionary, for his optimistic and positive outlook, and always standing beside me throughout my career and for being there at every step of the way to help me in this remarkable feat.

Hearty indebtedness to my mother and my in-laws for their constant emotional support and motivation.

Earnest gratitude to Professor Bisen, Retired VC (Jiwaji University, Gwalior, India)—a visionary academician—for guiding me in the right direction.

Overwhelming thankfulness to Dr. Rajesh Malik, who has been my mentor and an exceptional teacher.

Gratefulness to Dr. Akshara Gupta, HOD (Radiodiagnosis) and Dr. J. S. Sikarwar, superintendent, Jay Arogya Hospital (JAH), Gwalior, India for their professional guidance and encouragement.

Special thanks to Dr. Pankaj Yadav for his time and efforts in guiding and reviewing this book for me.

I would extend a deep personal thanks to the following people:

- To Dr. Ratnesh Jain for his time and efforts in preparing line diagrams for this book.
- To Dr. Sapna Somani, Dr. Mohinder Mehta, and Dr. Vipin Goyal who provided me sonographic images despite their busy schedule as private practitioners.
- To Dr. Shimanku Maheshwari Gupta, MD (Gynecology), for her inputs in the respective sections.
- To my seniors and colleagues: Dr. Lovely Kaushal, Dr. Amit Jain, Dr. Batham, Dr. Megha Mittal, Dr. Rajesh Baghel, Dr. Manohar, Dr. Purnima, Dr. Shiv, Dr. Sanyukta Ingle, and Dr. Yogesh for their generous guidance—given whenever required.
- To Dr. Saumya Mishra, SR, Sion Hospital, Mumbai for her contribution in preparing the thyroid and scrotum chapters.
- To Dr. Vivek Soni, Dr. Bhavya Shree (JR-3), Dr. Sandeep, and Dr. Manoranjan (JR-2) for assisting in formulating case reports and providing images from the department.
- To Trapti Nigam for technical assistance.

I would acknowledge and appreciate all the authors and editors whose books, journals, and websites I have gone through since my medical residency days and without which this book would never have come to fruition.

Immense thanks to Joana Koster, publisher, Taylor & Francis Group, CRC Press; Shivangi Pramanik, Assistant Commissioning editor (Medical); and her editorial assistant Mouli Sharma who green lighted this book; and Bala Gowri and Graphics team, Lumina Datamatics.

About the Author

Dr. Swati Goyal, DMRD, DNB is currently assistant professor, Department of Radiodiagnosis, at Government Medical College & Hospital, Bhopal, India, presently on deputation to Gajra Raja Medical College (GRMC) and Jay Arogya Hospital (JAH) Gwalior, India. She is simultaneously pursuing her PhD in medical sciences from Jiwaji University, Gwalior, India. She received her MBBS degree from Government Medical College (GMC), Amritsar, India. After completing residency from GMC and Maharaja Yashwant Rao Hospital (MYH), Indore, India she underwent training in Bhopal and was awarded DNB degree by National Board of Examinations (NBE) in New Delhi, India. She has served as senior resident in Chirayu Medical College, Bhopal and the All India Institute of Medical Science (AIIMS), Bhopal before joining GMC as an assistant professor.

She is a life member of Indian Radiological and Imaging Association (IRIA) and corresponding member of European Society of Radiology (ESR); she has undergone modular training in the revised national TB control programme (RNTCP) from Indore and has attended various state-level and national-level conferences. Her various research papers have been published in both national and international journals.

She has been contributing medical write-ups for an eminent newspaper *Times of India* and regularly writing articles pertaining to medical field on her Facebook page.

She is associated with Sonography Project *Spandan* based on mother and child health and *Dhanvantri project* initiated by the government for primary health facilities.

PART I

USG Physics

Ultrasound Physics

INTRODUCTION

Ultrasound waves are defined as sound waves of high frequency that are inaudible to the ear. These are *longitudinal* waves that propel in a direction parallel to that of wave propagation in a medium.

High-frequency sound waves are inaudible to humans in the range of 2–20 million cycles per second (2–20 MHz)—this is the range of a diagnostic ultrasound.

Sound audible to humans is <20 KHz
Ultrasound is >20 KHz
Speed of sound in air is 330 meters per second
Speed of sound in fat is 1,450 meters per second
Speed of sound in soft tissue is 1,540–1,580 meters per second
Speed of sound in bone is 4,080 meters per second

Principle of sonography

BASED ON PULSE-ECHO PRINCIPLE

Pulses of high-frequency sound waves are transmitted to the patient. Echoes returning from various tissue boundaries are detected. The received echo produces an ultrasound image (Figure 1.1).

Electricity converted into sound—Pulse
Sound converted into electricity—Echo
If more sound is received back—suggestive of stronger reflector—whiter image
If less sound is received back—suggestive of weaker reflector—blacker image

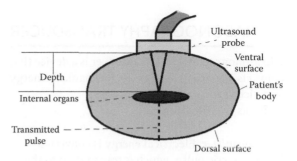

Figure 1.1 Illustrating principle of ultrasound.

Frequency: The number of cycles per second; measured in Hz (Hertz).
Wavelength: The distance between two consecutive waves. It depends on the frequency of waves and speed of propagation in the medium through which it is passing. It is inversely proportional to frequency.
Bandwidth: Range of frequencies produced by the transducer.
Pulse length: Small number of cycles in a pulse.

INSTRUMENTATION

1. *Transmitter*: Sends voltage to energize the transducer.
2. *Transducer*:
3. *Receiver*: To detect and amplify weak signals and send them to display It controls the dynamic range and time-gain compensation (TGC).
4. *Display*: To present the USG image/data in a form suitable for analysis and interpretation.

The transducer's input is communicated to scanner through a cable and the data can be visualized on the monitor.

Following are the ways through which spatial information can be displayed:

A mode: **A**mplitude mode; it is used for ophthalmic purposes
B mode: **B**rightness mode (gray scale, real time); it is used for routine sonography
M mode: **M**otion mode; it is used to measure the heart rate

ULTRASONOGRAPHY TRANSDUCER

Ultrasonography (USG) transducer is a device that converts electrical energy to mechanical energy and vice versa.

It has two functions:

1. *Transmitter*: Electrical energy is converted to acoustic pulse, which is transmitted to the patient.
2. *Receiver*: Receives reflected echoes. Weak pressure changes are converted to electrical signals for processing.

It is based on the principle of piezoelectricity.

Ultrasound pulses generated by transducer are propagated, reflected, refracted, and absorbed in tissues to provide useful clinical information.
Transducers (scanning probes) are the costliest part of any ultrasound unit.

Types of transducers

The shape of the scans from different transducers is different (Figure 1.2).

1. Curved array convex transducer: Wider fan-shaped image
   Useful for all body parts except echocardiography
   Large versions for general abdomino-pelvic and obstetrics scan
   Small high-frequency curved array scanners for transvaginal, transrectal scans
2. Linear array: Rectangular shape
   Most useful for small and superficial parts such as thyroid, testicle, and breast
   Vascular, musculoskeletal, and obstetric applications
3. Phased array sector scanner: Triangular fan shaped
   Used in cardiac examination through intercostal scanning

Selection of transducers

The thickness of transducer (usually 0.1–1.0 millimeters) determines its frequency (inversely proportional).
Each transducer is focused at a particular depth.
Penetration of the ultrasound diminishes with an increase in frequency.
Higher the frequency, shorter the wavelength, and better the resolution.
Frequencies from 7.5 to 15 MHz are used for superficial vessels and organs such as thyroid

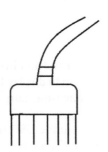
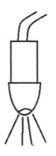
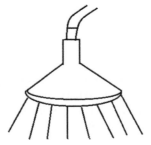

Rectangular image from linear array transducer

Narrow fan-shaped image from sector transducer

Wide fan-shaped image from convex transducer

Figure 1.2 Illustrating various types of transducers.

and breast lying within—1–3 centimeters of the surface.

Frequencies of 2–5 MHz are required for deeper structures in abdomen and pelvis, that is, >12–15 centimeters from the surface.

High frequency—better spatial resolution, greater attenuation, and poor penetration.

High frequencies →
- Broadens the bandwidth
- Reduces the quality factor (Q)
- Shortens the spatial pulse length (SPL)

Specialized transducers

1. Endovaginal probes for early obstetric and gynecologic problems.
2. Endorectal probes for prostate imaging.
3. Intraoperative/laparoscopic—it is used to insert through the laparoscopic port in the abdominal wall to enter into the abdominal cavity and retro peritoneum.

REAL-TIME ULTRASOUND

Real-time imaging systems are those that have frame rates fast enough to allow movement to be followed (>16 frame rates/second). For fast-moving structures such as heart, high frame rates are beneficial.

Types:

1. *Mechanical scanners*: Single-element transducer is mechanically moved to form images in real time. It is obsolete nowadays.
   - Oscillating transducer
   - Rotating wheel transducer
2. *Electronic array*: Transducers do not move but are activated electronically to cause ultrasound beam to sweep across the patient. It is most frequently used now.

CONSTRUCTION OF A TRANSDUCER

Piezoelectric crystal element: Located near the face of a transducer.

Outside electrode: Grounded to protect the patient from shock. Its outer surface is coated with a water-tight electrical insulator.

Inside electrode: Abuts against a thick backing block; absorbs the sound waves transmitted back into the transducer.

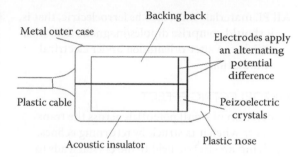

Figure 1.3 Illustrates construction of ultrasound transducer.

Backing block (Damping): Made of tungsten and rubber powder in epoxy resin.
- Absorbs the sound waves transmitted back into the transducer
- Shortens the pulse duration and pulse length (SPL)
- Increases axial resolution
- Widens the bandwidth and reduces the quality factor (Q)

Housing-strong plastic: Acoustic insulator of rubber/cork that prevents sound from passing into the housing (Figure 1.3).

Diagnostic transducers: Have damping material—wide bandwidth, low Q

Therapeutic transducers: Without backing material—narrow bandwidth

Piezoelectric crystal

Piezoelectric effect (PE) crystal is the main component of a transducer (located near the transducer's face).

Has the unique ability to respond to the action of an electric field by changing the shape (strain). Strain is the deformity of crystal (into different shapes) when voltage is applied to the crystal.

Have the property of generating electric potentials when compressed.

Naturally occurring PE materials—quartz, Rochelle salts, tourmaline.

Artificial PE materials—ferroelectrics—lead (Plumbium) zirconate titanate (PZT), barium lead titanate, lead metianobate, and polyvinylidene fluoride (PVDF).

Synthetic materials are good both at transmitting and receiving sound waves, whereas naturally occurring crystals are better at doing one or the other.

All PE materials must also be ferroelectric, that is, it should comprise dipoles/magnetic domains, which can alter orientation under electrical stimulation.

PIEZOELECTRIC EFFECT

Generation of small potentials across the transducer when it is struck by returning echoes.

Applying an electric field to the crystal leads to realignment of the internal dipole structure causing lengthening/contracting of the crystal. Hence, electrical energy is converted into kinetic/mechanical energy.

CURIE TEMPERATURE

The temperature above which a crystal loses its PE properties/polarization. Heating PE crystal above the Curie temperature reduces it to a useless piece of ceramic. Therefore, transducers should never be autoclaved.

Q FACTOR (QUALITY FACTOR OR MECHANICAL COEFFICIENT K)

Determines how effectively the transducer changes electrical voltage to sound.
High Q factor is associated with longer SPL.

ULTRASOUND GEL

Fluid medium that provides a link between the transducer and the patient's surface.

Coupling agent that transmits ultrasound waves to and from the transducer by eliminating the air between the transducer and the skin surface. (At a tissue–air interface, more than 99.9% of beam is reflected, so none of them is available for imaging.)

Components:

- Water
- Ethylene diamine tetra acetic acid (EDTA)
- Propylene glycol
- Carbomer
- Trolamine

Plain water is not a standard coupling agent as it tends to run away and evaporate from the body. It should be used only when nothing else is available. Oil, if used for a long time may damage the equipment and also stains the clothes.

Daily wipe the transducer after each examination. Put disposable gloves over the transducer in infectious patients such as HIV infected or with open wounds to prevent other patients from getting infected.

Bone absorbs ultrasound much more than soft tissues; therefore, ultrasound energy can reach only till the surface of the bone and not in the areas behind it, which appears black (acoustic shadowing).

Air reflects almost the entire energy of an ultrasound pulse coming through tissues, leading to blackness behind the gas bubble. Hence, sonography is not suitable for examining tissues containing air such as healthy lungs.

RESOLUTION

Contrast resolution

Depicted by different shades of gray in the image.
Improved by narrowing the dynamic range and using the contrast agent.

Temporal resolution

For a moving structure as in obstetrics and echocardiography
Also known as frame rate (number of images displayed per second)
Affected by depth and propagation speed
Improved by
- Reducing depth
- Narrowing the image sector
- Reducing the line density
- Switching off the multifocal

Spatial resolution

Determines the quality of sonographic image.
Determines the ability to differentiate two closely spaced objects as distinct structures (Figure 1.4).

Considered in three planes:

1. *Axial resolution*: Ability to separate structures *one over the other along* (*parallel*) the axis of the USG beam
   - Determined by pulse *length* (wavelength * number of cycles per pulse)
   - High transducer frequency provides higher image resolution
   - Most important

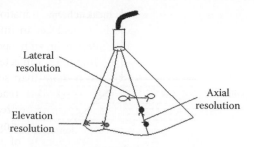

Figure 1.4 Depicting types of resolution.

Improved by
- Reducing SPL
- Damping
- Thin transducer elements
- High frequency
2. *Lateral resolution*
  In the plane *perpendicular* to beam axis and parallel to the transducer
  Ability to separate structures *side by side at the same depth*
  Determined by the *width* of USG beam
3. *Azimuth/elevation resolution*
  Determined by the slice thickness in the plane perpendicular to both beam and the transducer.
  Determined by the thickness of the USG beam.

NORMAL IMAGING

Echogenicity: Depends on density of structure, number, and type of reflectors within it and its interaction with the sound beam
Anechoic: Completely black without any echoes
Hypoechoic: Low-level echoes, less gray than the surrounding parenchyma
Isoechoic: Mid-level echoes similar to the surrounding parenchyma
Hyperechoic: White with high-level echoes
Echotexture: Depicted by different shades of gray
Homogenous: Similar shades of gray
Inhomogenous/heterogeneous: Different shades of gray in a tissue

Hence, echogenicity and echotexture are two distinct entities and tissues should be interpreted on both the parameters, for example, liver can be homogenous in echotexture with raised echogenicity, suggestive of diffuse fatty infiltration.

Orientation of probe

A marker should be pointed toward right during transverse scanning and towards the patient's head during longitudinal scanning.

Fresnel zone: Near zone
Fraunhofer zone: Far zone—(distal to focal point where sound beam diverges)

Time-gain compensation

It is one of the cardinal controls in the ultrasound unit. Echoes returning from deep structure are much weaker and severely attenuated than those from structures close to the transducer (stronger echoes).

Simply increasing the gain cannot settle this problem.

In order to compensate for signal loss from the far field, adjustment of sensitivity at each depth is required. This is possible with TGC, leading to uniform brightness at all depths for any solid organ, for example, liver.

Duty factor

Time spent to generate a pulse
Time spent sending signals/time spent receiving signals
Fraction of time, the transducer is actually on
Usually <1% for diagnostic ultrasound

Acoustic impedance

Resistance exerted by the medium to the propagation of sound through it

Density of medium×Velocity of sound in that tissue

Acoustic interface

Formed when sound waves pass from tissues with different impedances

Soft tissue–air interface (interface with large difference in acoustic impedance) reflects almost the entire beam, and thus there is no propagation of sound. This explains the inability of ultrasound to penetrate the air-filled lung and bowel. It also stresses the utility of coupling agent (gel) between the patient's body and the transducer.

Soft tissue–bone interface also reflects a major portion; hence, one should avoid ribs while scanning the liver.

Soft tissue–fat interface transmits relatively strong echoes, and hence helps in organ outlining.

INTERACTION WITH TISSUES

Reflection: Depends on the angle of incidence and acoustic impedance of tissue.

Angle of incidence: Angle between the sound beam and the reflecting surface.

Higher the angle less is the amount of reflected sound.

Specular reflector: If the acoustic interface is smooth and large.

Sound is reflected as a mirror reflects light, if insonated at 90 degrees.

For example, diaphragm, endometrium, and wall of fully distended urinary bladder.

Diffuse reflector: Multiple small interfaces of organs scatter echoes in all directions (Figure 1.5).

Refraction: Bending of waves when it passes from one medium to another (different speed of sound in different mediums) (Figure 1.6).

Angle of incidence is not 90 degrees.

Its frequency remains same, but wavelength changes.

Absorption: When a sound beam travels, some of its energy is converted into heat.

High absorption occurs with high frequency.

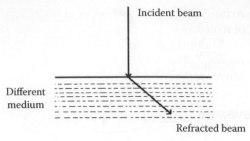

Refraction

Figure 1.6 Illustrates refraction of sound beam.

Deeper we go, more energy is lost, and image quality deteriorates.

Thus, low-frequency transducer has more depth penetration.

Scatter: Some of the echoes scatter nonuniformly in all the directions instead of reflecting back.

Attenuation: Combination of all the interactions.

Reduction in intensity of sound waves as it passes through tissues.

Causes absorption, scattering, and reflection of sound beam.

Proportional to the insonating frequency.

High-frequency probe—rapid attenuation and less penetration.

Attenuation value of

Water	0 (Zero) attenuation
Soft tissue	0.7
Bone	5
Air	10

IMAGING PITFALLS

1. Many artifacts suggest the existence of structures not actually present
   - Reverberation artifacts and comet tail artifacts
   - Refraction artifacts
   - Side-lobe artifacts
2. Some artifacts may clear off the real echoes from display or conceal information; crucial pathologies may be missed
   - Inappropriate adjustments of system gain and TGC settings
   - Imprudent selection of transducer frequency
   - Insufficient scanning angles
   - Inadequate penetration
   - Poor resolution

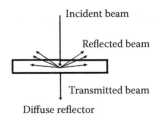

Diffuse reflector

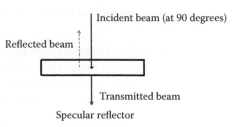

Specular reflector

Figure 1.5 Depicts specular and diffuse reflectors.

3. Artifacts that modify size, shape, and position of structures
   * Multipath artifacts
4. Acoustic shadowing and enhancement
5. Mirror artifacts

Reverberation artifacts

It arises when the USG signal reflects repeatedly between highly reflective interfaces near the transducer.

May give an erroneous notion of solid structures in areas where only fluid is present.

However, it is beneficial in recognition of surgical clips (special type of reflector).

Can be eliminated by changing the scanning angle to avoid the parallel interfaces contributing to the artifact.

Comet tail (Ring down) artifacts

Dirty shadowing with small bright *tail* behind closed interfaces seen

* Behind air bubbles.
* In the wall of gallbladder (GB) in adenomyomatosis.
* Behind puncture needle, if their angle to USG beam is approximately 90 degrees.

Comet tail is caused by reverberation between two closely spaced objects with discrete echoes posterior to the reflector.

Ring down is caused by acoustic impedance difference with enhancement posterior to the reflector.

Refraction

Bending of path of sound beam lead results in duplication of image in an unexpected and misleading location (simulated image).

Can be minimized by increasing the scan angle so that it is perpendicular to the interface.

Side lobe

Most of the energy is generated along the central axis by a transducer. Some low-intensity energy is also emitted from the sides of the primary beam that may create an impression of debris in fluid-filled structures.

Can be reduced by repositioning or changing the transducer.

Acoustic shadowing

Reduction in intensity of ultrasound (black zone) deep to a strong reflector (such as gas or foreign body) or extensive absorption in bones.

Useful for diagnosing calcifications, stones, or foreign bodies.

Limits the examination of areas behind gas/bones.

Acoustic enhancement

Structures that attenuate USG beam less than the surrounding tissues lead to too bright echoes behind them (Figure 1.7)

Usually seen in cystic lesions as illustrated in mainly Chapter 2,6,and 10

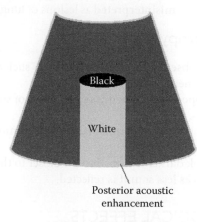

Black

White

Posterior acoustic enhancement

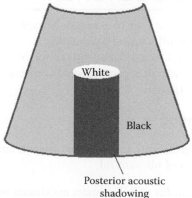

White

Black

Posterior acoustic shadowing

Figure 1.7 Depicting enhancement and acoustic shadowing.

Overpenetration

Echoes may be seen within normal fluid-filled structures such as bladder as they do not attenuate the USG pulses. Change the direction of the transducer.

Partial volume effect

If an ultrasound beam strikes a cyst smaller than the beam's cross section, cyst may show echoes inside and may be misinterpreted as a solid lesion.

Multipath artifacts

Creation of complex echo paths that decelerates the return of echoes to the transducer.

Results in display of the echo at an inappropriate location in the image.

Mirror artifacts

Surface of lung acts as a mirror. Structures of liver seen above the diaphragm (a strong smooth reflector) may be misinterpreted as lesions of lung.

Anisotropy

Usually observed in fibrous structures such as tendons, nerves, and bones.

Their appearance depends on the angle of sound waves.

If probe is held perpendicular to the direction of fibers, they appear bright.

They look darker if transducer is closer to the fibers as less sound is reflected.

BIOLOGICAL EFFECTS

Tissue heating: Due to absorption; used in physiotherapy ultrasound machines.

Cavitation: Occurs due to interaction of sound waves with microscopic, stabilized gas bubbles in the tissues.

Streaming

Two significant indices for measurement of bioeffects of ultrasound

Thermal index (TI): Evaluates maximum increase in temperature

Mechanical index (MI): Calculates cavitation effect of ultrasound

Both TI and MI should be <1 for obstetric sonography.

Pulse Doppler should not be used often, unless indicated.

Exposure time of fetus should be limited, according to as low as reasonably achievable (ALARA) principle.

Exposure of fetus to USG will be unsafe above 41 degrees.

CHAPERONE

A person who acts as a witness for both the patient and the medical practitioner during a medical examination or procedure.

The purpose is to provide reassurance and emotional support to a patient undergoing any procedure.

It also safeguards the doctor from an allegation of indecent behavior.

As per General Medical Council (GMC) guidelines

> Wherever possible you should offer the patient the security of having an impartial observer (a chaperone) present during an intimate examination (especially torso, breast, genitalia, and rectum). This applies whether or not you are of the same gender as the patient.

Chaperones need not be medically qualified. However, they should be conversant with procedures, so as to raise concerns about a doctor, if necessary. They could be a member of staff or a relative or friend of the patient or a third party of the same sex as the patient.

SUGGESTED READINGS

1. T. S. Curry and J. E. Dowdey, *Christensen's Physics of Diagnostic Radiology*, 4th ed., Wolter Kluwer, Philadelphia, PA, 1990.
2. J. L. Ball and T. Price, *Chesneys' Radiographic Imaging*, 6th ed., Wiley-Blackwell, Oxford, UK, 1995.
3. R. F. Farr and P. J. Allisy-Roberts, *Physics for Medical Imaging*, 2nd ed., Saunders Ltd., Edinburgh, UK, 2007.

4. P. E. S. Palmer, *Manual of Diagnostic Ultrasound*, World Health Organization, Geneva, Switzerland, 1995.

5. World Health Organization (WHO) and World Federation for Ultrasound in Medicine and Biology, *Manual of Diagnostic Ultrasound: Volume 1 & 2*, illustrated reprint edition, H. T. Lutz, E. Buscarini, and P. Mirk (Eds.), Geneva, Switzerland, 2013.

6. C. M. Rumack, S. Wilson, J. W. Charboneau, and D. Levine, *Diagnostic Ultrasound: 2-Volume Set*, 4th ed., Elsevier Health-US, Philadelphia, 2010.

PART II

Abdominal USG

Liver

INTRODUCTION

Anatomy

SEGMENTAL ANATOMY

Liver is divided into left and right lobe and various segments depending on the vascular supply. It has a dual blood supply from the portal vein and the hepatic artery, both directing the blood toward the liver. Three hepatic veins drain the blood from the liver into IVC, exhibiting a trident appearance on USG.

Left hepatic vein: Divides left lobe into medial and lateral segments.
Middle hepatic vein: Separates left and right hepatic lobe, also separated by gallbladder (GB) fossa; courses within the main lobar fissure.
Right hepatic vein: Divides right lobe into anterior and posterior segments.

Quadrate lobe: Medial segment of left hepatic lobe. Located between round ligament and GB fossa.
Caudate lobe: First segment of liver; bounded anteriorly by ligamentum venosum and posteriorly by IVC. It has its own blood supply and drainage. Should not be mistaken for a lymph node.

Glisson's capsule: Surrounds the liver and is thickest around the porta hepatis and IVC.

VASCULAR ANATOMY

Main Portal vein: Divides into right and left portal vein.

Right portal vein has anterior and posterior division.
Left portal vein has medial and lateral divisions.

They supply blood to the liver in their related segments (Figure 2.1 and Table 2.1).

Porta hepatis: Site at which portal vein, common bile duct (CBD), and hepatic artery are located within peritoneal fold called the hepatoduodenal ligament.

In utero, umbilical vein in liver divides into left and right.

Left umbilical vein: Connects directly to left portal vein. After birth, it becomes fibrous cord (Ligamentum teres/Round ligament). Ascends along the falciform ligament. Divides left lobe into medial and lateral segments.
Right umbilical vein (Ductus Venosus): Shunts blood directly into the IVC. After birth, it collapses and becomes ligamentum venosum.

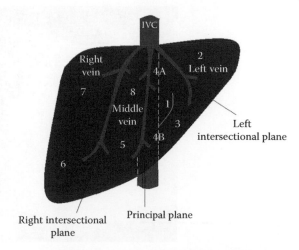

Figure 2.1 Illustrates segmental anatomy of liver.

Table 2.1 Illustrates Couinaud's segmental anatomy of liver

Segment 1	Caudate lobe
Segment 2	Lateral segment left lobe (superior)
Segment 3	Lateral segment left lobe (inferior)
Segment 4 (A&B)	Medial segment left lobe
Segment 5	Anterior segment right lobe (inferior)
Segment 6	Posterior segment right lobe (inferior)
Segment 7	Posterior segment right lobe (superior)
Segment 8	Anterior segment right lobe (superior)

Other ligaments

Coronary ligament: Right layer of the falciform ligament

Left triangular ligament: Left layer of the falciform ligament

Right triangular ligament: Most lateral portion of the coronary ligament

Bare area: The posterosuperior region of the liver, which is not covered by peritoneum

Protocol

Usually convex transducer (3.5 MHz) is used.

Nil by mouth except water for 8 hours before examination in adults and two to 3 hours in infants. In acute cases, immediate scanning may be required.

Patient should be scanned in supine, left oblique, and left lateral decubitus positions. Patient should be scanned in axial, sagittal, and oblique planes, including subcostal and inter-costal scanning.

Indications

1. Hepatomegaly
2. Right upper quadrant (RUQ) pain
3. Jaundice
4. Suspected liver abscess
5. Suspected liver mass and metastasis
6. Ascites
7. Trauma

Normal findings

Size: Usually <15 centimeters in midclavicular line.

Eye-balling technique: Liver extending below the lower pole of the right kidney is suggestive of hepatomegaly.

Reidel's lobe: Extension of the right lobe of liver, which is a normal variant.

Beaver tail liver: Sliver of liver, a variant where an elongated left lobe surrounds the spleen.

Echogenicity

Echogenicity of Pancreas > Liver ~ Spleen > Kidneys (cortex > medulla)

Homogenous parenchyma with thin-walled hepatic veins and bright reflective portal veins (Figure 2.2)

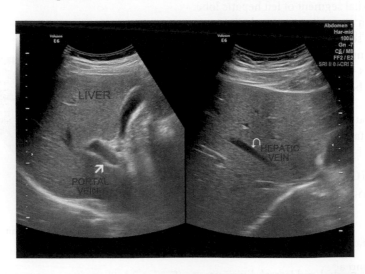

Figure 2.2 Depicting bright reflective portal vein walls and thin nonreflective hepatic vein walls.

PATHOLOGIES

Hepatitis

Hepatitis → Inflammation of liver due to varying etiologies.

ACUTE HEPATITIS

- Liver may appear normal.
- Tender hepatomegaly.
- Diffusely reduced/altered echogenicity.
- Increased brightness of portal triad (Periportal cuffing)—Starry sky pattern (Figure 2.3).
- Thickened edematous GB wall.

CHRONIC HEPATITIS

Liver may appear normal or reveal coarse echotexture with reduced echogenicity and diminished brightness of portal triad.

Cirrhosis

End-stage parenchymal disease.

- Coarse echo pattern secondary to nodularity and fibrosis. Micro- (<1 centimeter) and macronodules (up to 5 centimeters) may be seen
- Hepatomegaly in early stages and shrunken liver in advanced cases (Figure 2.4)
- Ascites
- Enlarged caudate lobe (width of *C/RL*-caudate lobe/right lobe >0.65 is suggestive of (S/o) cirrhosis)
- Splenomegaly
- Dilated portal vein
- Reduced vascular markings with decreased attenuation

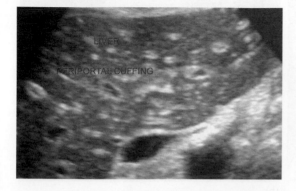

Figure 2.3 Depicting altered liver echotexture and periportal cuffing suggestive of hepatitis.

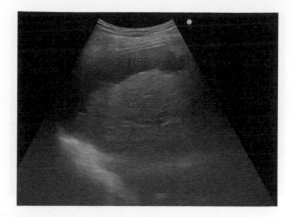

Figure 2.4 Depicting shrunken, coarse echotexture of liver with ascites.

Micronodular: Most commonly by alcohol
Macronodular: By chronic viral hepatitis

Causes of cirrhosis:

- Chronic hepatitis B & C
- Alcohol
- Nonalcoholic steato hepatitis (NASH)
- Autoimmune
- Genetic and inherited disorders
- Certain medications

Infective lesions

LIVER ABSCESS (PYOGENIC)

Cystic, septated complex lesion with irregular thick walls, ragged margins, and echogenic debris within.
Comet tail artifacts (dirty shadowing) may be seen if air is present in it.
Mature purulent abscess, in nature, is more cystic with debris.
Immature abscess may appear hypoechoic and solid in nature.

AMOEBIC ABSCESS

Well-defined round to oval hypoechoic lesion with low-level echoes. Caused by *Entamoeba histolytica*. May become heterogeneous in advanced infective cases (Figure 2.5).

SUBPHRENIC ABSCESS

Well-defined crescentic area between the liver and the right hemidiaphragm. Septa with debris may be seen on ultrasound.

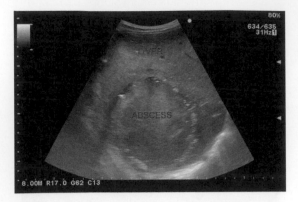

Figure 2.5 Depicting advanced amoebic liver abscess.

ECHINOCOCCAL (HYDATID) CYSTS

Caused by *Echinococcal granulosus*
Definitive host—dog
Intermediate host—sheep, cattle, humans

Three layers:

Pericyst: Outermost—connective tissue capsule
Ectocyst: External membrane ~1 millimeter thick, which may calcify
Endocyst: Innermost—germinal layer

Varying presentations (Figure 2.6a and b)

- Simple cyst with multiple daughter cysts (cyst within a cyst appearance—honeycomb appearance)

- Cysts with detached endocyst secondary to rupture (Water lily sign)
- Calcified mass/peripheral calcified lesion
- Honeycomb appearance due to septations

USG is helpful in monitoring the treatment response. Positive treatment response is suggested by reduction in size, increase in echogenicity, and calcification of cyst wall.

Fatty liver

Fatty liver: Seen as raised echogenicity with hepatomegaly (Figure 2.7a and b).
  Diminished portal vein wall visualization.
  Poor penetration of the posterior liver.
Mild: Minimal raised echogenicity.
Moderate: Raised liver echogenicity with slightly impaired visualization of diaphragm and vessel border.
Severe: Markedly raised echogenicity with poor visualization of diaphragm and vessel border.
Focal fatty deposits—(Focal hepatic steatosis):
  Focal areas of raised echogenicity in rest of the normal liver parenchyma.
Focal fatty sparing: Hypoechoic masses within an echogenic fatty liver.
Focal fatty changes are usually seen
  - In the medial segment of the left lobe of liver
  - In the region anterior to porta hepatis
  - Near the falciform ligament
  - Dorsal left lobe
  - Caudate lobe

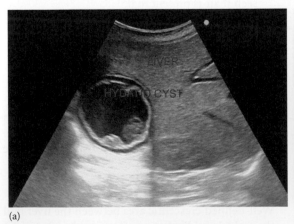

(a)

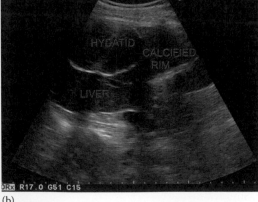

(b)

Figure 2.6 **(a)** and **(b)** Depicting hydatid cyst in liver.

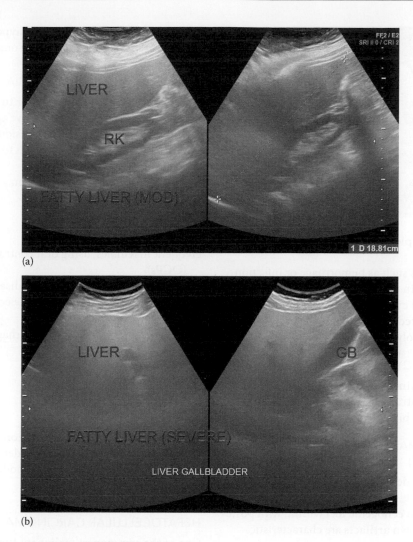

Figure 2.7 **(a)** and **(b)** Depicting fatty liver.

Hepatic vessels are normal and not displaced by fatty changes on Doppler study (lack of mass effect).

Seen as *geographical configuration* (map-like liver).

Fatty changes are commonly seen in diabetics, alcoholics, patients on exogenous steroids, certain drugs (chemotherapy, amiodarone, methotrexate), and IV hyperalimentation.

Fatty infiltration may resolve.

Focal hepatic lesions

1. Simple cysts
2. Peribiliary cysts
3. Hemangiomas
4. Biliary hamartomas
5. Focal nodular hyperplasia (FNH)
6. Hepatic adenoma
7. Biliary cystadenomas and carcinomas
8. Fibrolamellar carcinoma (FLC)
9. Hepatocellular carcinoma (HCC)
10. Metastases
11. Intrahepatic cholangiocarcinoma
12. Hematoma, infective lesions

SIMPLE CYSTS

Incidental, asymptomatic.

Well-defined, thin-walled anechoic lesion with posterior acoustic enhancement (Figure 2.8).

Sometimes may contain septations.

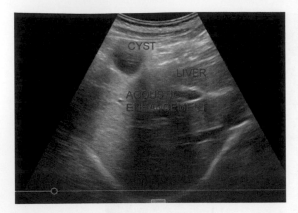

Figure 2.8 Depicting simple liver cyst.

Complications such as hemorrhage or infection may result in pain.

Multiple small cysts, usually <2–3 centimeters seen scattered throughout the liver parenchyma in polycystic liver disease.

PERIBILIARY CYSTS

Small (<2 centimeters) cysts, discrete, or clustered noticed centrally within the porta hepatis, paralleling the bile ducts and portal veins.

BILIARY HAMARTOMAS (VON MEYENBERG COMPLEXES)

Multiple, well-defined, tiny, nodular hypoechoic lesions.

Multiple bright echogenic foci within, with posterior ring down artifacts are characteristic.

HEMANGIOMA

Most common benign tumor of the liver.

Usually <3 centimeters, homogenously echogenic (Figure 2.9).

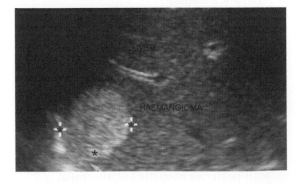

Figure 2.9 Depicting hyperechoic hemangioma.

May be heterogenous with central hypoechoic areas and thick echogenic borders in some cases.

FOCAL NODULAR HYPERPLASIA

Second most common benign liver tumor.

Common in females of reproductive age group.

Well-defined hyper to isoechoic lesion with a central scar, sometimes difficult to differentiate from adjacent normal liver.

Highly vascular central scar and may show spoke wheel pattern on Doppler.

HEPATIC ADENOMA

Frequent in females, using oral contraceptive pills (OCPs).

Associated with glycogen storage disease type 1.

Heterogeneous lesion with variable echogenicity seen.

Has propensity to undergo hemorrhage and malignant degeneration.

BILIARY CYSTADENOMAS

Middle-aged females.

Multilocular cystic mass.

Tends to recur after subtotal excision.

Can develop into malignant cystadenocarcinoma, manifesting with thick mural nodules and septae.

HEPATOCELLULAR CARCINOMA

One of the commonest malignant tumor.

Associated with cirrhosis and chronic viral hepatitis.

Occur in three forms—solitary, multinodular, and diffuse infiltrative (Figure 2.10).

Portal vein/hepatic vein (IVC) invasion is associated with poor prognosis.

Increased flow due to neovascularity and arteriovenous shunts.

FIBROLAMELLAR HEPATOCELLULAR CARCINOMA

Rare, seen in young patients.

Better prognosis.

Large, solitary, slow-growing mass with calcifications and central fibrotic scar.

Not associated with cirrhosis (c.f. hepatocellular carcinoma [HCC]).

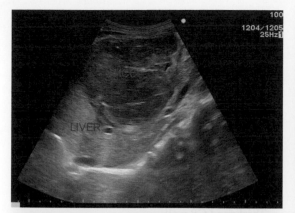

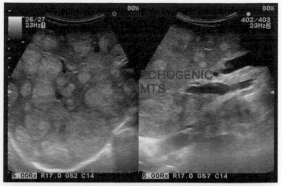

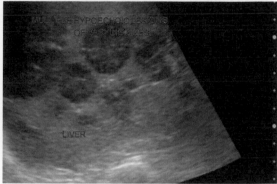

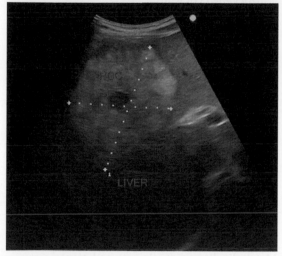

Figure 2.11 Depicting multiple liver metastasis (hyperechoic and hypoechoic) of varying sizes.

Figure 2.10 Depicting varying presentation of heterogeneous hepatocellular carcinomas.

METASTASES

Usually multiple, but may be rarely single.
Multiple, solid echogenic nodules with surrounding hypoechoic halo of varying sizes, giving *target sign* or *bull's eye sign* are suggestive of metastases (Figure 2.11).

Hyperechoic metastases

- Adenocarcinoma of colon
- Gastrointestinal tumors
- Renal cell carcinomas
- Carcinoid tumors
- Choriocarcinoma
- Islet cell tumor

Hypoechoic metastases

- Breast carcinoma
- Lung carcinoma
- May be from gastric, esophageal, and pancreatic cancers

Calcific metastases

- Mucinous adenocarcinomas (colon)

Cystic metastases

- Cystadenocarcinoma of ovary and pancreas
- Mucinous carcinoma of colon
- Necrotic colorectal metastases
- Neuroendocrine tumors

Diffuse infiltrative metastases

- Often confused with chronic liver disease
- Seen in breast and lung cancer; malignant melanoma

Pseudocirrhosis: Complication of treated (on chemotherapy) hepatic metastases, especially those of carcinoma breast.

Radiologically simulates liver cirrhosis with volume loss, caudate lobe enlargement, and capsular retraction.

INTRAHEPATIC CHOLANGIOCARCINOMA

Presents with painless jaundice.

Single, well-defined, and irregular hypoechoic mass often associated with capsular retraction.

Dilated intrahepatic bile ducts seen, which terminate at the level of tumor.

Thrombotic invasion of veins is rare (c.f. HCC).

HEMATOMA—H/O TRAUMA

Extracapsular: Echo-free or complex cystic lesion outside the liver capsule.

Subcapsular: Echo-free or complex cystic lesion between the capsule of the liver and the underlying liver parenchyma, curvilinear shaped usually compressing the liver parenchyma.

Parenchymal: Echo-free or complex cystic lesion in the liver parenchyma.

May be associated with lacerations, irregularly shaped hypoechoic lesions extending up to the capsular surface.

Posterior segment of right lobe is most commonly involved site in blunt trauma.

D/D biloma and abscess.

Miscellaneous

- Congestive hepatomegaly—seen due to congestive heart failure. Enlarged liver with dilated hepatic veins. Normal diameter of hepatic vein is up to 7–9 millimeters. Respiratory variation of IVC not seen. Associated with pleural effusion (Figure 2.12).
- Calcified granuloma from prior infective lesions, most commonly tuberculosis (Figure 2.13).

Pediatric section

NEONATAL HEPATITIS

Liver infection before the age of 3 months.

On USG—Diffuse hepatomegaly
    Thickened GB wall
    Abscess (if bacterial origin)

Biliary atresia—Ghost triad of GB:

- Absent/small GB <1.5 centimeters length
- Irregular/lobular contour
- Indistinct wall with lack of complete echogenic mucosal lining

Triangular cord sign: Echogenic cord-shaped density just cranial to portal vein bifurcation.

CAUSES OF CIRRHOSIS IN CHILDREN

Hepatitis
Cystic fibrosis
Metabolic diseases (toxin accumulation)
Biliary atresia

INFANTILE HEMANGIOENDOTHELIOMA

Single/multiple solid masses of varying echogenicity
Multiple tortuous vessels seen both within and at the periphery of the mass

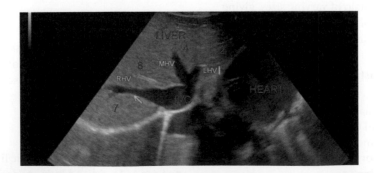

Figure 2.12 Depicting congestion of hepatic veins and IVC. Trident of hepatic veins also describes segmental anatomy of liver.

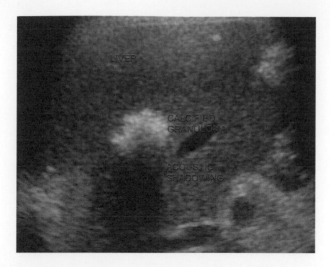

Figure 2.13 Depicting calcified granuloma of TB with acoustic shadowing.

Celiac axis, hepatic artery, and hepatic veins appear dilated due to severe arteriovenous shunting
Infraceliac aorta appears small

MESENCHYMAL HAMARTOMAS

Rare, multiseptated cystic mass
<2 years age group

HEPATOBLASTOMA

Most common primary liver tumor of childhood
    <3 years: Heterogeneous vascular mass with scattered calcifications, mostly in the right lobe of the liver. High serum alpha-fetoprotein (AFP).

UNDIFFERENTIATED EMBRYONAL SARCOMA

Malignant mesenchymoma. Rare; 6–10 years age group.
Rapidly growing, large, heterogeneous with central necrosis and cysts.
Normal serum AFP levels.

METASTASES

Diffuse infiltration of the liver or multiple nodules.
From neuroblastoma, Wilm's tumor, leukemia, or lymphoma.

Figure 2.43 Depicting calcified granuloma of TB with acoustic shadowing.

Celiac axis, hepatic artery, and hepatic veins appear dilated due to severe arteriovenous shunting. Infrarenal aorta to appear small

MESENCHYMAL HAMARTOMAS

Rare; multiseptated cystic mass
<5 years age group

HEPATOBLASTOMA

Most common primary liver tumor of childhood
<2 years. Heterogeneous vascular mass with scattered calcifications, mostly in the right lobe of the liver. High serum alpha-fetoprotein (AFP)

UNDIFFERENTIATED EMBRYONAL SARCOMA

Malignant mesenchymoma. Rare; 6–10 years age group.
Rapidly growing, large, heterogeneous with central necrosis and cysts
Normal serum AFP levels.

METASTASES

Diffuse infiltration of the liver or multiple nodules.
From neuroblastoma, Wilm's tumor, leukemia, or lymphoma.

3

Gallbladder

INTRODUCTION

USG should be performed after a minimum of 4 hours of fasting, since ingestion of fatty food stimulates the contraction of the gallbladder (GB). GB also contracts after administration of cholecystokinin.

Anatomy

GB lies in the inferior margin of the liver in the same anatomic plane as the middle hepatic vein (MHV) (Figure 3.1).

Interlobar fissure extends from the origin of the right portal vein (RPV) to the GB fossa and used as a landmark.

Parts of GB—Fundus, body, and neck (Hartmann's pouch, a common location for impaction of stones).

Valve of Heister: Located in cystic duct, prevents it from collapsing/overdistending.

Hartmann's pouch: Outpouching of GB neck.

Normal GB wall thickness—3 millimeters.

>5 millimeters is definitely abnormal.

Normal GB demonstrates posterior acoustic enhancement.

Overdistended GB: If transverse diameter >4 centimeters and longitudinal diameter 9–10 centimeters. May be known as gallbladder hydrops, if measurement exceeds the normal.

Reexamine after a fatty meal. If no contraction occurs, look for obstruction in the cystic duct and common bile duct (CBD) by stones, clots, ascariasis, and external compression by lymph nodes or neoplasm.

The contracted GB appears thick walled and may obscure luminal or wall abnormalities.

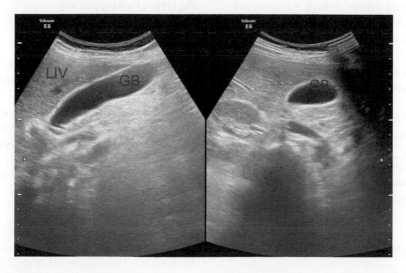

Figure 3.1 Depicting normal gallbladder and liver in different sections.

Variants of gallbladder

1. Ectopic GB
2. Septate GB
3. Duplication of GB
4. Phrygian cap (GB fundus folded over the body)

In patients with jaundice

Distended GB is suggestive of CBD obstruction (intra-/extraluminal). Look for intrahepatic biliary radicles (IHBRs).

Nondistended GB suggests nonobstruction of CBD or obstruction above the level of cystic duct.

Curvoisier's sign—Patients presenting with painless jaundice and palpable gallbladder (RUQ mass) are unlikely to have stones in GB. Pancreatic/biliary neoplasm should be presumed as a cause until proven otherwise.

PATHOLOGIES

Gallstones (Cholelithiasis)

Risk factors: Fat, fertile, female, pregnancy, diabetes, and so on.

USG

- Mobile, echogenic foci giving posterior acoustic shadowing.
- Stones change in position within the lumen as the patient moves in comparison to nonshadowing polyps, which are constant in position. Calculus may sometimes get impacted at neck.

Scanning with the patient in lateral decubitus or upright position allows the stone to roll within the GB.

Wall-Echo-Shadow (WES) complex: In a GB filled with stones, GB *wall* is first visualized in the near field. Followed by the bright *echo* of the stone. Followed by the acoustic *shadowing*. Commonly mistook for either rib shadow or bowel gas (Duodenum lies posterior to GB and may cause shadowing).

Bile sludge/sand/microlithiasis

Sludge is a precipitate of bile solutes.

Predisposing factors—pregnancy, rapid weight loss, prolonged fasting, critical illness, long-term total parental nutrition (TPN).

Reversible GB sludge/stone formation (Pseudolithiasis) has been reported after administration of ceftriaxone therapy (third-generation cephalosporins), which may disappear after 1 month of discontinuation of the drug and can prevent unnecessary cholecystectomy.

On USG:

- Amorphous, low-level echoes within the GB in a dependent part without acoustic shadowing (Figure 3.2)
- Tumefactive sludge/sludge balls may mimic stones (but are without shadowing) or tumors
- Lack of internal vascularity
- Mobile (change position very slowly with change in patient's position)
- GB wall is normal

It may disappear after treatment of the cause or may progress to form gallstones. Follow-up scans are required.

Hepatisation of gallbladder: GB lumen is completely filled with tumefactive sludge with GB simulating liver parenchyma, leading to nonvisualization of GB on USG. However, normal liver parenchyma demonstrates color flow on Doppler imaging, whereas GB will not.

Acute cholecystitis

USG finding spectrum

1. Stones in GB (neck or cystic duct)
2. Thickened GB wall (>3 millimeters) (Figures 3.3 and 3.4)
3. GB wall edema, striated with pockets of fluid
4. Distended GB (>4 centimeters diameter)
5. Positive sonographic Murphy's sign—Probe tenderness over the GB
6. Increased vascularity of the GB wall
7. Pericholecystic fluid collections
8. Sludge

Gangrenous cholecystitis: Sloughed membranes appearing as linear intraluminal echoes.

Perforation: Disruption of GB wall with adjacent collection.

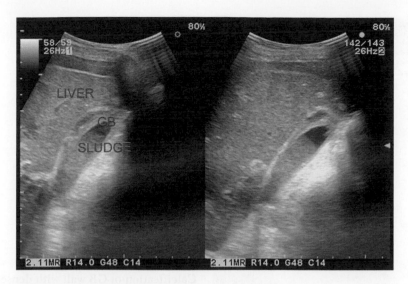

Figure 3.2 Depicting sludge in the GB lumen.

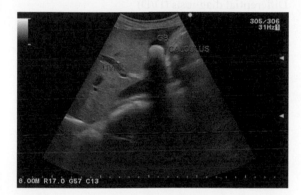

Figure 3.3 Depicting echogenic calculus in the lumen.

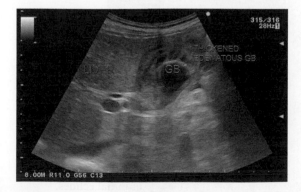

Figure 3.4 Depicting thickened GB wall in a patient with cholecystitis.

Emphysematous cholecystitis: Intraluminal air as bright echogenic foci with dirty shadowing.

Xanthogranulomatous cholecystitis: A rare inflammatory disease of GB with focal/diffuse wall thickening, intramural nodules, stones, and loss of fat plane with adjacent liver parenchyma. Difficult to differentiate from malignancy.

Acalculous cholecystitis

Usually found in critically ill patients with major surgery, severe trauma, sepsis, diabetes, and atherosclerosis.

GB distension, wall thickening, internal sludge, and pericholecystic fluid in terribly ill patients.

Miscellaneous

Causes of nonvisualization of GB (Figure 3.5)

1. Nonfasting patient. Minimum 4–6 hours fasting required for adequate distension of GB.
2. Contracted GB full of calculi/fully calcified GB giving acoustic shadowing.
3. GB in unusual position.
4. H/o cholecystectomy.
5. Congenital hypoplasia/aplasia of GB—very rare.
6. Hepatization of GB.

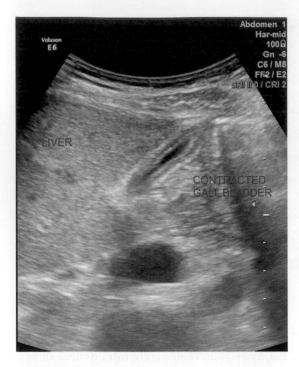

Figure 3.5 Depicting thickened and contracted GB wall.

Causes of GB wall thickening.

Systemic
1. Congestive heart failure (CHF)
2. Renal failure
3. Hypoalbuminemia (ascites)
4. End-stage cirrhosis

Inflammatory
1. Cholecystitis
2. Cholangitis
3. Hepatitis
4. Pancreatitis

Neoplastic
1. GB adenocarcinoma
2. Metastasis

Miscellaneous
1. Adenomyomatosis
2. Mural varicosities
3. Ascites

Porcelain gallbladder

Calcification of GB wall with dense posterior acoustic shadowing, female predominance

High risk of GB carcinoma

Differential diagnosis (D/D)
1. *Gallstones*: WES complex is absent in porcelain GB.
2. *Emphysematous cholecystitis*: Dirty shadowing is absent in porcelain GB.

Polyps

Multiple, nonshadowing, and nonmobile lesions adherent to the GB wall (c.f. mobile gallstones) (Figure 3.6).

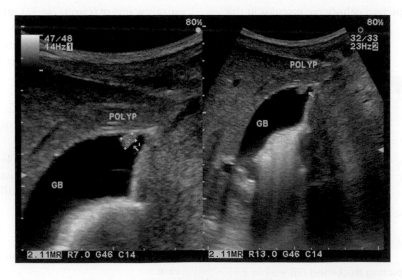

Figure 3.6 Depicting nonshadowing, nonmobile polyp in the GB lumen.

Adenomyomatosis

- Benign.
- Can be focal or diffuse.
- Thickening of GB wall with internal cystic spaces or debris (echogenic) creating comet tail artifacts simulating the appearance of cut kiwi fruit in diffuse adenomyomatosis.

Gallbladder carcinoma

- Vascular heterogeneous mass replacing the normal GB fossa.
- Trapped stones may be noted.
- GB may be obliterated and adjacent liver may be infiltrated (Figure 3.7).
- CT scan is recommended to detect its extensions.

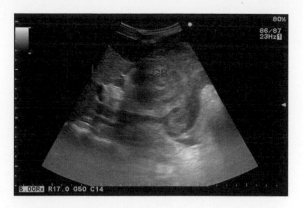

Figure 3.7 Depicting GB lesion infiltrating the adjacent liver.

4

Biliary Tree

INTRODUCTION

In biliary terminology, *proximal* denotes the portion of the biliary tree *closer to liver*, whereas *distal* end denotes the part *closer to the bowel*.

The right and left hepatic ducts, that is, first-order branches of common hepatic duct (CHD) are routinely visualized on USG.

Normal CHD—5 millimeters.

Normal common bile duct (CBD)—5–6 millimeters. Increase in 1 millimeter per decade noticed after the age of 60, which may increase up to 10–12 millimeters in postcholecystectomy patients.

CBD is visualized as an anechoic duct just above the portal vein at porta hepatis.

Dilated IHBR's are seen as central and peripheral tubules parallel to portal venules.

PATHOLOGIES

Choledocholithiasis (CBD stones)

Primary: *De novo* formation of stones in the biliary ducts.

Secondary: Migration of stones from GB (or after cholecystectomy).

On USG:

- Echogenic lesions with posterior acoustic shadowing.
- Small stones may lack good acoustic shadows and appear as bright linear echogenicity (Figure 4.1).

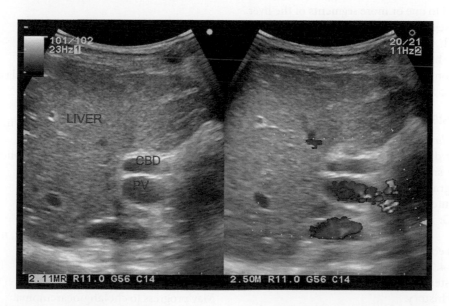

Figure 4.1 Depicting dilatation of CBD.

D/D's

1. Blood clot (hemobilia), air (pneumobilia), papillary tumors, biliary sludge.
2. Surgical clips due to previous cholecystectomy—short length, high degree of echogenicity, absence of GB, lack of ductal dilation.

MIRIZZI SYNDROME

- Stone impacted in the cystic duct with surrounding edema.
- Dilatation of biliary ducts to the level of the common hepatic duct.

Cholangitis

ACUTE CHOLANGITIS
USG

- Dilatation of the biliary tree (Figure 4.1).
- Choledocholithiasis and sludge.
- Bile duct wall thickening.
- Hepatic abscesses.

Presents with fever, RUQ pain, and jaundice (*Charcot's triad*).

Recurrent pyogenic cholangitis
On USG

- Dilated ducts filled with sludge and stones, confined to one or more segments of the liver. Lateral segment of the left lobe is most often involved.
- Chronic biliary obstruction, stasis, and stone formation lead to recurrent episodes of acute pyogenic cholangitis.

ASCARIASIS

Ascariasis lumbricoides, a parasitic round worm, commonly due to low hygiene levels. It is active within the small bowel and may enter the biliary tree retrogradely through the ampulla of Vater causing acute biliary obstruction.
    On USG:

- Parallel echogenic lines within the bile ducts (Figure 4.2). The appearance is similar to biliary stent, which should be excluded on clinical history.

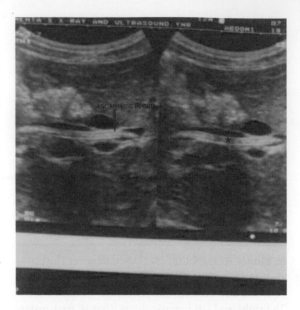

Figure 4.2 Depicting ascariasis in the dilated CBD just above the portal vein.

- On transverse view, the round worm surrounded by a duct wall gives target appearance.
- Movement of worm during the scan facilitates the diagnosis.

HIV cholangiopathy

Pain, cholestasis, markedly elevated serum alkaline phosphatase (SAP) and normal bilirubin levels.

On USG:

- Bile duct wall thickening.
- Focal strictures and dilatations.
- Diffuse GB wall thickening.
- Dilated CBD due to stenosed papilla of Vater.

Sclerosing cholangitis

Chronic inflammatory process involving the biliary tree.
Strongly associated with ulcerative colitis (70%).
Biliary strictures and cholestasis.

On USG:

- Irregular bile duct wall thickening, narrowing the lumen.
- Focal strictures and dilatations.

May progress to cholangiocarcinoma.

Cholangiocarcinoma

Neoplasm arising from any part of biliary tree.
Classified based on the anatomical location:

1. Hilar (Klatskin's)—60%
2. Distal—30%
3. Intrahepatic (Peripheral)—10%

Approximately 90% of these are adenocarcinomas.

HILAR CHOLANGIOCARCINOMA

Present with jaundice, pruritus, and elevated cholestatic liver parameters. Increased SAP or gamma glutamyl transpeptidase (γGT) levels.
On USG:

- Dilatation of higher order IHBDs with nonunion of the right and left hepatic ducts.
- Tumor extension into segmental ducts bilaterally precludes resection.
- Narrowing of either portal vein leads to compensatory increased flow in the accompanying hepatic artery. May lead to atrophy of the involved lobe.
- Lymphadenopathy in porta hepatis, hepatoduodenal ligament, extending to celiac, superior mesenteric, and peripancreatic nodes.
- Usually metastasizes to liver and peritoneal surfaces.

CT/MRI recommended for preoperative assessment.

DISTAL CHOLANGIOCARCINOMA

Most common type.
On USG: Varying presentations

- Polypoid tumor seen as intraductal mass with expanding duct.
- Focal irregular ductal constriction and duct-wall thickening.
- Hypoechoic, hypovascular, ill-defined mass, infiltrating other structures.

INTRAHEPATIC

Least common location for cholangiocarcinoma.
Second most common primary malignancy of the liver.
Poor prognosis.

On USG:

- Mass forming type—Heterogeneous, hypovascular solid mass, usually associated with capsular retraction.
- Periductal infiltrating type—narrowed or dilated ducts.
- May be seen as polypoid mass in the bile ducts, distending the lobar and distal ducts due to abundant mucin production.

Pediatric section

BILIARY ATRESIA

Ghost triad of GB—Absent/small GB <1.5 centimeters length.

Irregular/lobular contour.
Indistinct wall with lack of complete echogenic mucosal lining.

Triangular cord sign: Echogenic cord-shaped density just cranial to portal vein bifurcation.

CHOLEDOCHAL CYSTS

Congenital cystic dilations of biliary tree.
Todani's classification:

Type I: Focal/diffuse dilatation of extrahepatic bile duct (Figure 4.3)
Type II: True diverticulum of the bile duct
Type III: Choledochocele—dilatation of distal (intraduodenal) CBD
Type IVa: Multiple intrahepatic and extrahepatic biliary dilatations (IH + EH)
Type IVb: Cyst confined to extrahepatic biliary tree (EH)
Type V: Caroli's disease (cysts confined to intrahepatic biliary tree) (IH)

Recently type-VI choledochal cyst (cystic dilatation of the cystic duct) has been added in the classification.
ERCP/MRCP is recommended for further evaluation.

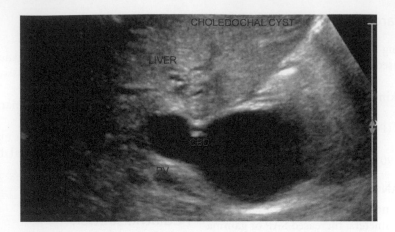

Figure 4.3 Depicting type-I choledochal cyst.

BILIARY RHABDOMYOSARCOMA

Children present with intermittent obstructive jaundice manifesting as hepatomegaly, abdominal pain and distension, weight loss, clay stools, and dark urine.

Heterogeneous cystic mass, usually in the intraductal location.

5

Spleen

INTRODUCTION

Anatomy

The average adult spleen measures
~12 × 7 × 4 centimeters (L × B × T) with an
average weight of 150 grams.

Normal adult spleen is convex superolaterally and
concave inferomedially.

It lies between the diaphragm and the fundus of
the stomach, with its long axis in the line of the
tenth rib.

Modest inspiration depresses the central portion
of left hemidiaphragm and spleen inferiorly for
easy visualization.

An oblique section along the intercostal space
avoids rib shadowing.

On USG, spleen has homogenous parenchyma with mid- to low-level echogenicity
(Figure 5.1).

Normal splenic vein measures up to 10 millimeters in diameter.

PATHOLOGIES

Splenomegaly

Mild to moderate: Infections such as TB, malaria,
fungal, protozoal, and so on
- Portal hypertension
- AIDS

Marked: Myeloproliferative disorders
- Leukemia, lymphoma
- Infectious mononucleosis
- Myelofibrosis

Cystic lesions of spleen (Figure 5.2)

1. *Infectious cysts*: Hydatid cysts (one of the least
   common site), may be calcified.
2. Posttraumatic pseudocyst.
3. *Epidermoid cysts*: Congenital.
4. *Intrasplenic pancreatic pseudocysts*: Associated
   with features of pancreatitis.

Figure 5.1 Depicting normal echotexture of
spleen.

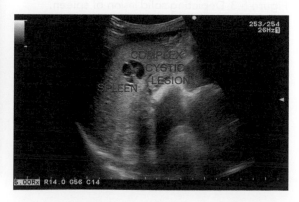

Figure 5.2 Depicting cystic lesion of spleen.

35

5. *Splenic abscess*: Complex cyst with irregular thick walls and debris. Dirty shadowing is seen if air is present. Follow-up after appropriate treatment is required.

The echoes from cholesterol and debris mimic a solid lesion.

Solid lesions of spleen (Figure 5.3)

1. *Granulomatous infections*: Focal, bright echogenic lesions with or without shadowing. Includes histoplasmosis, tuberculosis, and sarcoidosis.
   D/D—calcifications in the splenic artery.
2. *Primary malignancy*: Rare and includes primary lymphoma and angiosarcoma.
3. *Metastases*: May be hypo/hyper/mixed echogenic lesions.
   From malignant melanoma, carcinoma of breast, lung, and stomach.
4. *Hemangiomas*: Most common primary splenic tumor. Well-defined echogenic/mixed echogenicity. Usually small in size and benign.

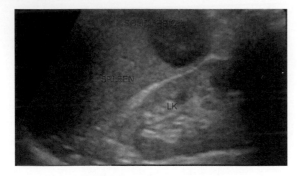

Figure 5.3 Depicting solid lesion of spleen.

5. *Infarct*: Peripheral, wedge-shaped hypoechoic lesion without vascularity and progression to hyperechoic lesions over time. Occur in children with vasculitis and sickle cell anemia.
6. Gaucher's disease.
7. Schistosomiasis.
8. *Candidiasis*: Wheel within wheel appearance.
9. *Miliary TB*: Innumerable tiny echogenic foci scattered diffusely.
10. *Trauma*: Subcapsular, pericapsular, and intraparenchymal hematoma.
11. *Gamma Gandy nodules*: Seen in portal hypertension.

Miscellaneous

Splenunculi: Accessory spleen—normal variant. Confused with enlarged lymph nodes.
  Usually seen near the splenic hilum with similar echogenicity as spleen.
  CT/Tc99m heat damaged RBCs can confirm the diagnosis.
Asplenia and *polypsplenia* are seen in patients with visceral heterotaxy.
Polysplenia: Bilateral left-sidedness. They have morphologically two left lungs, left-sided azygous continuation of IVC, biliary atresia, absent gallbladder (GB), gastrointestinal malrotation, and cardiovascular abnormalities.
Asplenia: Bilateral right sidedness. They have two morphologically right lungs, midline liver, reversed position of aorta and IVC, horseshoe kidneys, and anomalous pulmonary venous return.
Posttraumatic splenosis: Splenic cells may implant throughout the peritoneal cavity following splenic rupture, leading to multiple ectopic splenic rests.

6

Pancreas

INTRODUCTION

Anatomy

Nonencapsulated, retroperitoneal structure that lies in the anterior pararenal space between the duodenal loop and the splenic hilum.

Supplied by gastroduodenal artery (GDA) and splenic artery.

Length: 12.5–15 centimeters.

Parts: Head, uncinate process, neck, body, and tail.

Two ducts: Main pancreatic duct (MPD)—Duct of Wirsung—drains through *major* papilla.

Accessory pancreatic duct—Duct of Santorini—open into the duodenum at *minor* papilla.

USG: Normally, it has homogenously hyperechoic echotexture.

With aging and obesity, it becomes more echogenic as a result of fatty infiltration.

Anteroposterior (AP) dimensions of normal (Figure 6.1):

Head—Up to 3.0 centimeters.

Body—Up to 2.5 centimeters.

Tail—Up to 2.0 centimeters.

GDA lies anteriorly and common bile duct (CBD) lies posteriorly in the pancreatic head.

Normal variant

Sometimes the posterior half of pancreatic head reveals diminished echogenicity due to lesser fat content of ventral embryonic anlage. Can simulate a hypoechoic lesion and has to be differentiated by lack of biliary dilatation and absence of mass effect.

Technique

Patient preparation—Minimum fasting of 6 hours.

Erect/semierect position displaces gas-filled stomach or colon away from the pancreas.

If not possible, stomach distension with water also allows pancreatic visualization.

PATHOLOGIES

Acute pancreatitis

Causes: Most common are biliary tract calculi and alcohol abuse.

USG examination is more beneficial, 48 hours after the acute episode as the paralytic ileus resolves.

FOCAL

- Focal and hypoechoic enlargement of pancreas, usually head.
- Difficult to differentiate from neoplasm. Consider clinical severity and amylase/lipase correlation for acute pancreatitis.

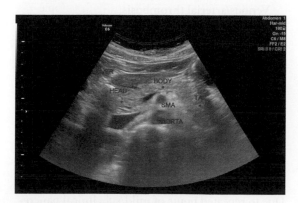

Figure 6.1 Depicting normal anatomy of pancreas and adjacent structures.

- Gradually tapering CBD.
- Usually seen in chronic alcoholics, but may also be caused due to adjacent inflammatory process such as penetrating peptic ulcer.

DIFFUSE

- Diffusely hypoechoic parenchyma and certain inhomogenities with increasing severity.
- Pancreatic duct may appear dilated.

MILD

- Normal on USG with abnormal clinical and laboratory findings.
- Reduced echogenicity and increasing size (due to edema and inflammation) are observed as the condition worsens (Figure 6.2).

Extrapancreatic manifestations:

1. Fluid collections in lesser sac, anterior pararenal space, and so on.
   Seen within 4 weeks from the onset of an acute attack with high incidence of spontaneous regression.
   Can be treated conservatively with serial sonography scans.
2. Ascites.
3. Thickened edematous gallbladder (GB) wall.
4. Pleural effusion (left sided).

COMPLICATIONS

1. *Pancreatic pseudocysts*
   Well-defined, walled-off pancreatic fluid collection that persists for at least 4 weeks from the onset of acute inflammation.

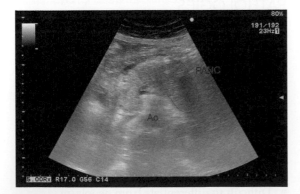

Figure 6.2 Depicting enlarged, hypoechoic pancreas in acute pancreatitis.

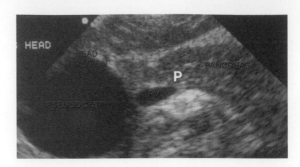

Figure 6.3 Depicting pseudocyst formation as a complication of acute pancreatitis.

4–6 weeks are required to form a wall composed of collagen and vascular granulation tissue.
On USG
- Well-defined, anechoic cystic structure (Figure 6.3). Debris may be seen if infected or hemorrhagic.
- May have calcified walls in chronic cases.
  May regress spontaneously or requires decompression if
  Persists >6 weeks.
  Size >6 centimeters.
  Complications such as infection, internal hemorrhage, and perforation occur.
  1. *Acute peritonitis*: May occur with rupture of pseudocyst into the peritoneal cavity.
  2. *Pancreatic abscess*: Thick-walled anechoic mass containing debris with bright echoes (reverberation artifacts) from gas bubbles.
2. *Vascular complication*
   Venous/arterial thrombosis.
   Pseudoaneurysm formation (portal vein/splenic artery).
3. *Pancreatic ascites*
   Due to slow leakage of pancreatic enzymes into the peritoneal cavity from disruption of MPD.
   Asymptomatic with enlarging abdomen.
   ERCP can detect the location of PD disruption.

Chronic pancreatitis

Progressive, irreversible destruction of the pancreas.
Due to repeated bouts of mild/subclinical pancreatitis resulting from high alcohol intake/biliary tract disease.

USG

- Heterogeneous echotexture of pancreas with patches of hypoechoic (due to inflammation) and hyperechoic foci (due to fibrosis and calcification).
- Calcifications due to intraductal calculi.
- CBD and pancreatic duct (PD) appears dilated (irregular dilatation).
- Pseudocysts that do not tend to resolve spontaneously.

Adenocarcinoma

Tumors arising in the *head* (70%)—Earlier present due to CBD obstruction.

Manifests with painless jaundice and palpable nontender GB.

Tumors in the *body and tail*—Later presents with weight loss, pain, jaundice, and vomiting when the gastrointestinal tract (GIT) is invaded by the tumor.

USG

- Poorly defined heterogeneous/homogenous hypoechoic mass in the region of pancreatic head (Figure 6.4).
- Hypovascular on Doppler imaging.
- Dilated PD >2–3 millimeters, may appear tortuous.
- CBD dilatation with abrupt termination is highly suggestive of malignancy.
- Thick echogenic sludge in CBD/Gallbladder.
- Double duct sign—Both CBD and PD are dilated.
- Compression, invasion, encasement of vascular structures.

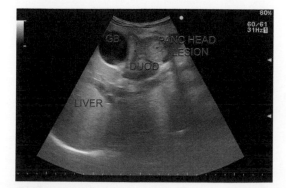

Figure 6.4 Depicting carcinoma pancreas infiltrating the adjacent duodenum.

- Small cystic areas due to necrosis may also be seen.
- Has poor prognosis.

D/D

1. Focal acute pancreatitis.
2. Focal mass associated with chronic pancreatitis.
3. Peripancreatic lymphadenopathy—Presence of echogenic septa between nodes.
4. Ampullary adenocarcinomas—Has better prognosis.

Endoscopic ultra sonography (EUS) combines endoscopy and high-resolution sonography.

Indicated in detection and staging of even small tumors, chronic pancreatitis, and morbidly obese patients but is highly operator dependent.

Cystic neoplasms of pancreas

MICROCYSTIC/SEROUS CYSTADENOMA

>60 years (granny's tumor): female preponderance, always benign.

USG

- Well-defined, lobulated, slightly echogenic, apparently solid but multicystic mass.
- Cysts <2 centimeters with a central stellate-shaped echogenic area (Scar).
- Pseudocapsule and septa of these tumors tend to be vascular.

MACROCYSTIC/MUCINOUS CYSTADENOMAS/ CYSTADENOCARCINOMAS

Frequently involves 40–45 years females (mommy's tumor).

- Well-circumscribed, uni/multilocular cystic lesions, usually cysts >2 centimeters in size.
- May be anechoic or echogenic containing debris or solid mural vegetations.
- Even the malignant ones have better prognosis.
- Surgical removal.

INTRADUCTAL PAPILLARY MUCINOUS TUMOR/NEOPLASM

M = F (same incidence in males and females).
Presents as recurrent pancreatitis.
Originates from MPD or its branches.

Segmental/diffuse dilatation of MPD with/without side-branch dilatation.

Branch type presents as a single or multicystic mass.

Communication with pancreatic duct differentiates it from other cystic neoplasms.

Best visualized on endoscopic retrograde cholangio pancreatography (ERCP)/(MRCP) magnetic resonance cholangio pancreatography.

Islet cell tumors: Rare—Functioning tumors include the following:

Insulinomas (B cell tumors)

Gastrinomas

Glucagonoma

VIPoma

Somatostatinoma

Carcinoid

On USG: Difficult to detect because of their small size

Usually well defined and hypoechoic without calcifications/necrosis

SOLID PAPILLARY EPITHELIAL NEOPLASMS

Young females (teenager's tumor).

Large well-defined encapsulated tumor with a propensity for hemorrhage and necrosis.

Pancreatic tail predilection.

Better prognosis.

Point to note: High *Amylase* levels in pseudocysts, acute pancreatitis, and low in serous cystic tumors.

Carbohydrate antigen (*CA 19-9*) levels high in ductal and mucinous cystic neoplasms.

Carcino embryonic antigen (*CEA*) increases in mucinous tumors and reduces in pseudocysts and serous cystadenomas.

Pediatric specific

PANCREATOBLASTOMA

Rare, invasive tumor in children. Heterogeneous solid, multilocular cystic areas with hyperechoic septae; mostly in the head of pancreas.

Associated with high alpha-fetoprotein (AFP).

CYSTIC FIBROSIS

Echogenic pancreas due to fatty replacement. Cysts <3 millimeters may also be seen.

NESIDIOBLASTOSIS

Diffuse echogenic enlargement of pancreas (tumor-like condition) due to diffuse proliferation of primitive ductal epithelial cells. Often associated with hypoglycemia and Beckwith–Wiedmann syndrome.

7

Genitourinary Tract, GUT

INTRODUCTION

Anatomy

- Left kidney usually lies—1–2 centimeters higher than the right. Extends from T12-L3 vertebrae usually.
- Normal kidney measures approximately 9–13 centimeters in length and 4–6 centimeters in width. Size of both the kidneys should not differ by >2 centimeters (Figure 7.1).
- Renal parenchyma is composed of
  Cortex: Usually less echogenic than the adjacent liver and spleen.
  Medullary pyramids: More hypoechoic than cortex.
- Echogenic renal sinus containing urine collecting system, blood vessels, fat, and fibrous tissue seen in the center of kidney.
- The kidney has a thin, fibrous true capsule. Perirenal fat lies outside this capsule, encased anteriorly by the fascia of Gerota and posteriorly by the fascia of Zuckerandl.

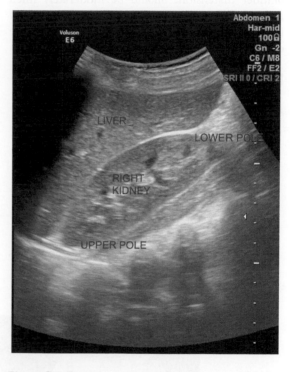

Figure 7.1 Depicting normal echotexture of right kidney in comparison to liver.

Vascular anatomy

Bilateral renal arteries arise from aorta at L1-2 vertebral body level.

Left renal vein is longer, passes between aorta and superior mesenteric artery (SMA) before entering into IVC.

Left gonadal vein drains into the left renal vein.

Right renal artery is longer, courses inferiorly, and passes posterior to IVC and right renal vein.

Left renal artery passes posterior to the left renal vein.

Four protective layers covering the kidney (inner to outer):

1. Fibrous capsule
2. Perirenal fat
3. Gerota's fascia
4. Pararenal fat

Ureters

30–34 centimeters long and 2–8 millimeters diameter. Nondilated ureter may not be visualized due to the overlying bowel gas. Normally, lie anterior to iliac vessels.

Bladder

Trigone is an area demarcated by the ureteric and urethral orifices within the bladder. The wall thickness of bladder depends on the degree of bladder distension. Should be moderately filled for proper visualization. Normal bladder capacity is ~400–500 milliliters. Postvoid scan should be done to rule out any lower urinary tract pathology.

Normal variants

Hypertrophied column of Bertin: Normal variant representing the unresorbed polar parenchyma. Sonographically, usually, seen at the junction of upper and middle thirds of the kidney.
Bordered by junctional parenchymal defect.
Indentation of renal sinus laterally.
Continuous with adjacent renal cortex.
It contains renal pyramids.
Generally <3 centimeters. May be misinterpreted for a small tumor. Presence of arcuate arteries by color Doppler (CD) differentiates it from a small tumor.

Renal hypoplasia: Kidney is small in size but otherwise normal.
Persistent fetal lobulation: Fetal kidney is normally lobulated. May persist as normal variant in adults.
Dromedary hump: Normal variant of contour of kidney due to splenic impression into superolateral border of the left kidney. It may simulate a renal mass but calyces and pyramids may extend into this pseudotumor.

PATHOLOGIES

Hydronephrosis

Dilated calyceal system and continuity of calyceal with renal pelvis differentiates it from cysts. Pelvi–calyceal system may dilate due to overhydration, overfilled urinary bladder (relieves after micturition), and pregnancy.

Grade1: Minimal splitting of pelvis—may be due to overfilled bladder.
Grade2: Mild—dilated pelvis and calyces.
Grade3: Moderate—both pelvis and calyceal system are dilated with mild parenchymal atrophy.
Grade4: Severe—markedly dilated pelvi–calyceal system with severe thinning of renal parenchyma (Figure 7.2).

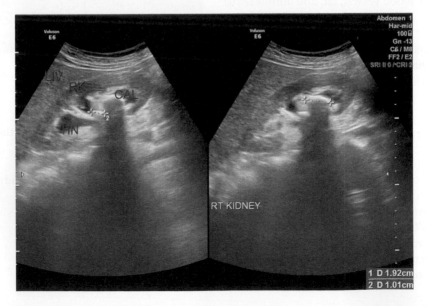

Figure 7.2 Depicting varying grades of hydronephrosis as mild.

(Continued)

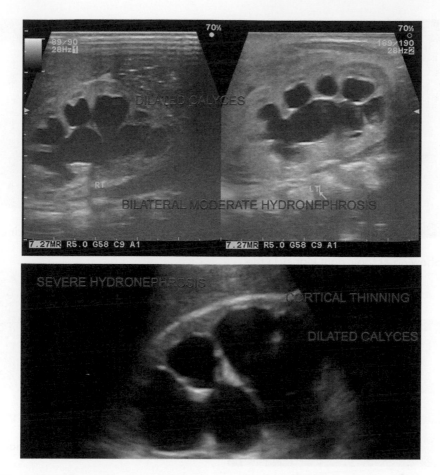

Figure 7.2 (Continued) Depicting varying grades of hydronephrosis as moderate and severe.

Congenital anomalies

RENAL DUPLICATION

Partial or complete duplication of the collecting system.

WEIGERT–MEYER RULE

The lower pole collecting system inserts into the bladder at the normal site, but intramural portion may be shorter than usual leading to vesicoureteric reflux (VUR).

The upper pole ureter inserts ectopically inferomedial to the site of normal ureteral insertion. Its orifice may be stenosed and obstructed.

Patients with complicated renal duplications may present with urinary tract infections, failure to thrive, hematuria, and symptoms of bladder obstruction.

Females with urethral insertion of the upper pole ureter below the external urinary sphincter may present with chronic constant urinary incontinence or dribbling.

ECTOPIC KIDNEY

Failure of kidney to ascend during embryologic development results in pelvic kidney.

Kidneys are small sized with reduced functioning.

Ureters are short (Figure 7.3).

If the kidney ascends too high, it passes through Bochdalek's foramen, results in thoracic kidney.

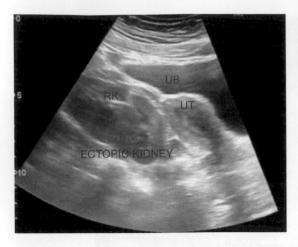

Figure 7.3 Showing ectopic right kidney in the pelvis.

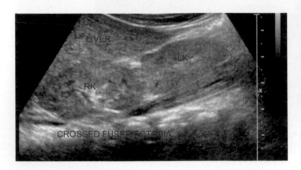

Figure 7.4 Illustrating normal right kidney cross fused with ectopic right kidney.

CROSSED FUSED ECTOPIA

Both kidneys are found on the same side.
Ectopic kidney will be fused to the other kidney (Figure 7.4).
Ureteric-vesical junction (UVJ) is normally located.

HORSESHOE KIDNEY

Lies anterior to the abdominal great vessels.
Fusion of lower poles with either functioning or fibrous isthmus.
Associated with pelvi-ureteric junction (PUJ) obstruction, VUR, and so on.
On sonography, kidneys are lower than normal with the poles projecting medially (Figure 7.5).
Hydronephrosis and calculi may be seen.

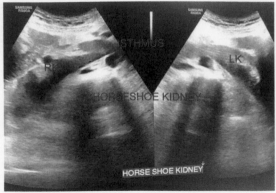

Figure 7.5 Illustrating horseshoe kidney.

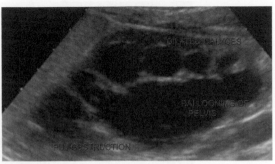

Figure 7.6 Illustrating PUJ obstruction.

PELVI-URETERIC JUNCTION OBSTRUCTION

M:F=2:1.
Left > Right.
On sonography, hydronephrosis up to the level of pelvi-ureteric junction.
Marked ballooning of the renal pelvis is present (Figure 7.6).

Infective lesions

ACUTE PYELONEPHRITIS

Usually kidneys appear normal. If abnormal, may show

- Altered echotexture
- Renal enlargement
- Loss of cortico-medullary differentiation

If focal, may appear as hypoechoic masses.
    Untreated or inadequately treated APN may lead to parenchymal necrosis with abscess formation.

Diabetics, immunocompromised, and patients with chronic debilitating diseases are at an increased risk.

On USG, round, thick-walled hypoechoic complex masses with internal mobile debris.

Sometimes gas with dirty shadowing may also be seen.

D/D

- Hemorrhagic/infected cysts
- Parasitic cysts
- Multilocular cysts/cystic neoplasms

Small abscess: Treated conservatively.
Large abscess: Requires per cutaneous drainage/ surgery.

PYONEPHROSIS

Purulent material in an obstructed collecting system
On sonography, hydronephrosis ± hydroureter
- Mobile debris (Figure 7.7)
- Gas with dirty shadowing may be seen
- Stones may be seen

CHRONIC PYELONEPHRITIS

Interstitial nephritis often associated with VUR.
On sonography

- Echogenic parenchyma with atrophy
- Dilated collecting system

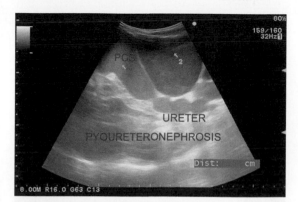

Figure 7.7 Depicting dilatation of pelvicalyceal system and ureter with enlarged kidney and echogenic debris suggesting pyoureteronephrosis.

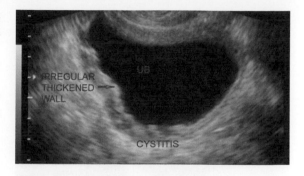

Figure 7.8 Depicting thickened and irregular bladder wall in a patient with cystitis.

CYSTITIS

Usually caused by *E. coli*.
Presents with bladder irritability and hematuria.
On sonography
- Diffuse irregular bladder wall thickening (Figure 7.8)
- Internal mobile echoes in the lumen may be seen

Calculi

RENAL CALCULI

Most common type of stone is calcium oxalate (60%–80%).

Three areas of ureteric narrowing where the stone may lodge:

1. Just past the PUJ
2. Where the ureter crosses the iliac vessels
3. At the UVJ (most common site as ureter has its smallest diameter of 1–5 millimeters here)

On sonography → echogenic foci with distal acoustic shadowing seen and proximal hydroureteronephrosis. Sometimes hydronephrosis may not be present suggesting nonobstructing calculi. Twinkling artifacts may be seen on Doppler.

Staghorn calculus—coral calculus—take the shape of renal pelvis resembling horns of a stag. Occur due to recurrent infection; usually composed of struvite (Magnesium, Ammonium, Phosphate [MAP]).

Entities that mimic renal calculi

- Renal artery calcifications
- Intrarenal gas
- Calcified sloughed papilla

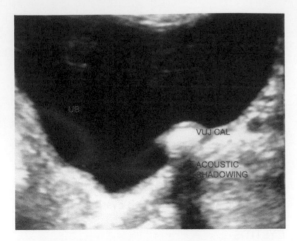

Figure 7.9 Showing a calculus at VUJ leading to upstream hydroureteronephrosis.

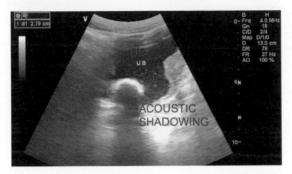

Figure 7.10 Illustrating two calculi in the urinary bladder lumen.

Ureteric calculi are difficult to visualize due to overlying bowel gas and the deep retroperitoneal location of ureters. However, it can be seen by applying pressure on the transducer (Figure 7.9).

Bladder calculi: Mobile, echogenic foci with distal acoustic shadowing. Thickened bladder wall and edematous ureteral orifice may be seen. *Jackstone calculus* is an irregular (resembles toy jacks and star anise sometimes) dense calculus with spicules radiating outward; usually composed of calcium oxalate dehydrate (Figure 7.10).

Renal cystic disease

1. *Cortical cysts*
   Simple
   Complex
2. *Medullary cyst*
   Medullary sponge kidney (MSK)
   Medullary cystic disease

3. Parapelvic cyst
4. Polycystic kidney disease (PCKD)–AR (autosomal recessive), autosomal dominant (AD)
5. Multicystic dysplastic kidney (MCDK)
6. Multilocular cystic nephroma (MLCN)
7. Acquired cystic kidney—in patients with dialysis
   In patients with renal cell carcinoma (RCC)
8. Associated with Von Hippel Lindau (VHL) syndrome, tuberous sclerosis (TS)

SIMPLE RENAL CYSTS

Incidence increases with ageing.

On sonography—Well-defined, imperceptible, anechoic, round/ovoid lesion with acoustic enhancement (Figure 7.11).

If small—No intervention is required. Regular follow-up required.

If large and symptomatic—Cyst puncture and sclerosis may be done.

COMPLEX RENAL CYSTS

Cyst containing internal echoes, septations, calcification, perceptible wall, and mural nodularity (Figure 7.12).

On imaging:

Infected cyst: Demonstrate thickened wall with debris-fluid level or gas in the cyst. Aspiration and drainage required.

Hemorrhagic cyst: Echogenic debris in the cyst. Follow-up by serial USG for interval changes required.

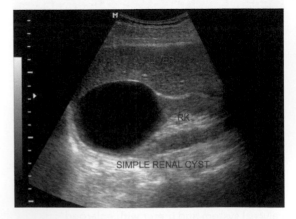

Figure 7.11 Shows thin-walled anechoic cyst at the upper pole of right kidney.

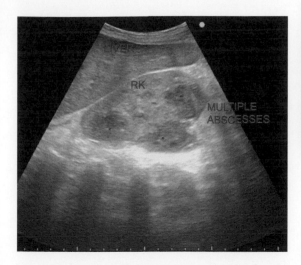

Figure 7.12 Showing multiple abscess with mobile echogenic debris.

Septation

<1 millimeter thin septa, smooth—likely benign.
>1 millimeter thick septa, irregularly thickened, or solid elements—malignant etiology.

Sonography is better than CT scan in defining the internal character of a cystic lesion.

PARAPELVIC CYSTS

On sonography

- Well-defined anechoic renal sinus masses
- Do not communicate with the collecting system
- May become infected/ hemorrhagic if internal echoes are seen in the cyst

D/D—Hydronephrosis—anechoic fluid-filled calices communicating with the renal pelvis.

MEDULLARY SPONGE KIDNEY

Dilated ectatic collecting tubules localized to the medullary pyramids. Multiple echogenic shadowing foci if nephrocalcinosis is present.

MEDULLARY CYSTIC DISEASE

Medullary cystic disease associated with progressive renal tubular atrophy.
On sonography—small echogenic kidney (nephronophthisis) with 0.1 to 1 centimeter medullary cysts at the corticomedullary junction.

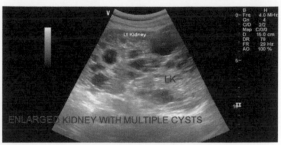

Figure 7.13 Illustrating multiple cysts of varying sizes in an enlarged polycystic kidney.

AUTOSOMAL RECESSIVE POLYCYSTIC KIDNEY DISEASE

On sonography—Massively enlarged echogenic kidney with lack of corticomedullary differentiation (CMD).

AUTOSOMAL DOMINANT POLYCYSTIC KIDNEY DISEASE

M = F

Bilateral cortical and medullary renal cysts (Figure 7.13)
S/S—Pain, hypertension, hematuria, and urinary tract infection (UTI)
Complications—Infection, hemorrhage, stone formation, rupture, and obstruction
Sonographically—Enlarged kidney with multiple bilateral asymmetrical cysts of varying sizes

MULTICYSTIC DYSPLASTIC KIDNEY

M = F

Small malformed kidney with multiple cyst and nonfunctional renal parenchyma.
If bilateral, incompatible with life.

On USG

Multiple noncommunicating cysts.
Absent in both normal renal parenchyma and renal sinus.

MULTILOCULAR CYSTIC NEPHROMA

Rare benign cystic neoplasm
On USG—Multiple noncommunicating cyst with a well-defined mass
D/D—Cystic RCC

Medical disease of genitourinary tract

Patients presenting with abnormal renal function tests especially serum creatinine levels are sent to USG department for initial screening test to rule out any mechanical obstruction or renal parenchyma abnormality.

Most common causes

1. *Acute tubular necrosis (ATN)*: May be normal/enlarged echogenic kidney. Suggest contrast enhanced computed tomography (CECT) (striated nephrogram) for further evaluation.
2. *Acute cortical necrosis (ACN)*: Initially the cortex is hypoechoic, gets calcified with time. CECT reveals cortical rim sign.
3. *Acute glomerulonephritis (AGN)*: Normal/markedly enlarged bilateral kidney with altered echotexture.
4. *Chronic glomerulonephritis (CGN)*: With progression, global symmetric parenchymal loss leading to small, smooth echogenic kidney and prominent central echo complex.
5. *Acute interstitial nephritis (AIN)*: Hypersensitivity reaction leading to enlarged echogenic kidney.
6. *Diabetes mellitus*: Most common cause of chronic renal failure (CRF).
   On USG
   - Reduction in size of kidney
   - Raised cortical echogenicity and preserved CMD
   - With progression to end-stage disease, kidneys become smaller, more echogenic and the medulla becomes as echogenic as the cortex. (Small shrunken kidneys with raised echogenicity) (Figure 7.14)

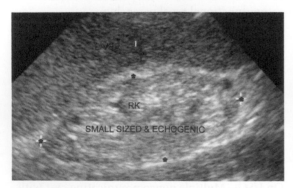

Figure 7.14 Illustrating echogenic shrunken kidney s/o advanced diabetic nephropathy.

7. *Amyloidosis*: Enlarged kidneys (in acute stages), later on which may reduce in size, demonstrates cortical atrophy, and raised echogenicity with progression.

Neoplastic lesion

RENAL CELL CARCINOMA

M:F = 2:1

50–70 years

Associated with smoking, hypertension, obesity, chemical exposure

Presentation—Flank pain, gross hematuria, and palpable renal mass

Histologic subtypes:

1. Clear cell carcinoma—70%–75% cases
2. Papillary carcinoma~15% cases
3. Chromophobe type~5% cases
4. Oncocytoma~2%–3% cases
5. Collecting duct/medullary tumors~1%

On USG, tumor may be solid iso/hypo/hyperechoic (Figures 7.15 and 7.16)

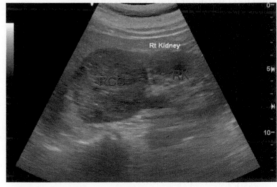

Figure 7.15 Illustrating solid tumor RCC.

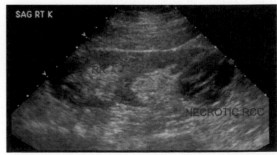

Figure 7.16 Illustrating necrotic RCC at lower pole.

- Cystic degeneration associated with necrosis and calcifications may be seen.
- Peripheral hypoechoic rim may be seen.

Four growth patterns of cystic variety of RCC

1. Multilocular cystic RCC with thick nodular septations
2. Unilocular cystic RCC—debris-filled cystic mass with thick, irregular walls
3. Necrotic RCC
4. Tumors originating in simple cyst

CECT is a better modality to diagnose renal carcinoma.

ROBSON'S STAGING

Stage 1: Tumor confined within the renal capsule.
Stage 2: Invasion of perinephric fat.
Stage 3: Regional lymphadenopathy or venous invasion (IVC).
Stage 4: Invasion of adjacent organs or distant metastases.

Stage 1 and 2 can be treated surgically. Stage 3 requires thrombectomy along with surgery. Stage 4 can be managed only palliatively.

TRANSITIONAL CELL CARCINOMA

Multifocal; Bilateral; M>F.
Associated with analgesic abuse, heavy smoking, exposure to carcinogens, cyclophosphamide.

RENAL TRANSITION CELL CARCINOMA

On USG:

- Hypoechoic renal sinus masses with or without associated proximal caliectasis.
- May extend into parenchyma with distortion of renal architecture, but maintained reniform shape.
  D/D—blood clots, fungus ball, and sloughed papilla.

URETERIC TRANSITIONAL CELL CARCINOMA

Usually involves lower third of ureter with proximal hydroureteronephrosis.

BLADDER TRANSITIONAL CELL CARCINOMA

Most common site—trigone, lateral, and posterior bladder wall.

On USG:

Focal nonmobile mass/urothelial thickening with or without calcifications.
70% cases are superficial and 30% are invasive.
D/D—Cystitis, wall thickening due to bladder outlet obstruction, adherent blood clot (clot changes its position with change in patient position and is avascular).

Cystoscopy and biopsy are necessary for diagnosis.

SQUAMOUS CELL CARCINOMA

Associated with chronic infection (schistosomiasis), irritation, stones, and leukoplakia.

ADENOCARCINOMA

Rare, associated with UTI.

LYMPHOMA

Usually non-Hodgkin's lymphoma. Present as

- Focal parenchymal—Solitary or multiple nodules.
- Diffuse infiltration—Disrupted renal architecture with preserved reniform shape.
- Direct invasion by retroperitoneal lymph node masses.
- Perirenal involvement seen as hypoechoic perirenal mass.

ONCOCYTOMA

On USG, iso/hypo/hyperechoic; usually well defined

- Central scar, necrosis, or calcifications seen
- Difficult to differentiate from RCC

ANGIOMYOLIPOMA

On USG, classic angiomyolipomas (AMLs) are hyperechoic relative to renal parenchyma. Prone to aneurysm formation and hemorrhage because vessels in AML lack normal elastic tissue.

Miscellaneous

COMPENSATORY HYPERTROPHY

Diffuse: Enlarged but otherwise normal kidney. Seen with nephrectomy, renal agenesis, renal atrophy, or dysplasia.

Focal: Large areas of nodular normal renal tissues in an otherwise diseased kidney as in reflux nephropathy; may mimic a solid renal mass.

ENLARGED KIDNEYS

1. Glomerulonephritis or pyonephritis (acute and subacute)
2. Lymphoma
3. Polycystic kidneys
4. Nephrotic syndrome
5. Metastases
6. Amyloidosis
7. Acute renal vein thrombosis

SMALL KIDNEYS

1. Chronic renal disease
2. Chronic pyelonephritis
3. Tuberculosis
4. Renal artery stenosis
5. Congenital hypoplasia
6. Infarction
7. Chronic glomerulonephritis
8. End-stage renal vein thrombosis

GENERALIZED THICKENING OF THE BLADDER WALL

1. Chronic cystitis
2. Prostatic obstruction
3. Urethral valves leading to chronic outlet obstruction
4. Schistosomiasis (associated with calcification)
5. Neurogenic bladder
6. Incomplete filling of bladder

LOCALIZED THICKENING OF BLADDER WALL

1. Polyp/neoplasm
2. Hematoma/blood clots due to trauma
3. Incomplete filling of the bladder
4. Infectious/inflammatory causes such as TB, and so on

ECHOGENIC LESIONS WITHIN THE BLADDER LUMEN

1. Calculus—Usually mobile, may be adherent
2. Polyp—Sessile or pedunculated
3. Foreign body, catheters
4. Blood clot/hematoma due to trauma (Figure 7.17)

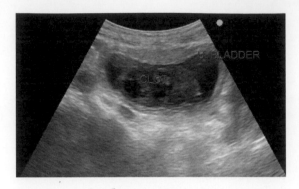

Figure 7.17 Depicting heterogeneous blood clot in the urinary bladder lumen, mimicking a tumor.

5. Air due to infection, fistula, or catheterization—reverberation artifacts seen
6. Sometimes an enlarged prostate/large uterine fibroid centrally at the base of bladder
7. Neoplasm

RENAL TRAUMA

1. *Minor injury*: Contusions, subcapsular hematomas, small cortical infarcts, and lacerations that do not extend into the collecting system.
2. *Major injury*: Lacerations that may extend into the collecting system.
3. Vascular pedicle injury.
4. Uretero-pelvic junction (UPJ) avulsion.

URETEROCELE

It is cystic dilatation of intramural portion of ureter. On USG, seen as cystic structure projecting into the bladder near VUJ. May be uni- or bilateral. May produce obstruction leading to recurrent UTIs.

NEUROGENIC BLADDER

Detrusor areflexia: Lower motor neuron lesion—on USG, appears as smooth, large capacity, thin-walled bladder extending high into the abdomen.

Detrusor hyperreflexia: Thick-walled, vertical, trabeculated bladder—associated with dilated upper tract and large postvoid residual volume.

BLADDER DIVERTICULA

Congenital: *Hutch* diverticula—Located postero-
laterally near the ureteric orifice.
Acquired: Due to bladder outlet obstruction.

USG

- Outpouching sac from the bladder.
- Neck is easily appreciated (Can be narrow or wide).
- Urine may be seen flowing into and out of the
  diverticulum. Debris may be seen (Figure 7.18).

URETERAL JET

This pattern is seen when the denser urine from the
ureter flows into the diluter urine in the bladder.
Ureteral jets flow in anteromedial direction. Can
be used to assess the patency of the ureter. Absence
of jet does not suggest obstruction but its presence
excludes complete obstruction (Figure 7.19).

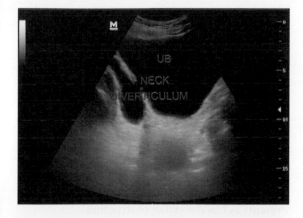

Figure 7.18 Illustrating urinary bladder diverticula.

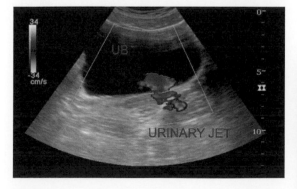

Figure 7.19 Illustrating urinary stream showing
color on Doppler.

Pediatric section

Infant kidney differs from the adult kidney in various aspects as the following:

1. Central echo complex is less prominent than
   renal parenchyma because of less peripelvic fat
   in infants.
2. Echogenicity of renal cortex is same as that of
   liver in a term child (c.f. Older children and
   adults in whom renal cortex is less echogenic
   than liver and spleen).
   Renal cortical echogenicity is higher than liver
   and spleen in very premature infants.
3. Medullary pyramids are larger and prominent in infants. May be mistaken for multiple cysts or dilated calyces. However,
   normal pyramids line up around the central
   echo complex in a characteristic pattern
   and hence can be differentiated from cysts
   (Figure 7.20).
4. Corticomedullary differentiation (CMD) is
   greater probably because of less overlying
   body fat.

PRUNE–BELLY SYNDROME (EAGLE–BARRETT SYNDROME)

Congenital absence or deficiency of the abdominal
    musculature
Hypotonic dilated tortuous ureters
Large bladder
Patent urachus
Bilateral cryptorchidism
Associated pulmonary hypoplasia may lead to
    Potter's syndrome and death

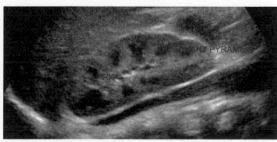

Figure 7.20 Illustrates normal infant kidney.

MEGACYSTIS–MICROCOLON MALROTATION INTESTINAL HYPOPERISTALSIS SYNDROME

Enlarged bladder, hydronephrosis, and hydroureter with microcolon, malrotation, and diminished to absent peristalsis of the bowel.

EXSTROPHY OF THE BOWEL

Pubic bones are far apart and expose the bladder and urethral mucosa.

Normal kidneys and ureters.

URACHAL ANOMALIES

Urachus is a tubular structure extending from the umbilicus to the bladder. It normally closes by birth and a remnant may be visible as a hypoechoic mass on the anterosuperior aspect of the bladder.

If it remains patent, urine may leak from the umbilicus.

If part of urachus closes, patent part may form urachal cysts, which may become infected.

If proximal portion of the urachus remains open, it forms a diverticulum-like structure from the dome of the bladder.

WILM'S TUMOR (NEPHROBLASTOMA)

Most common intraabdominal malignant tumor to occur in child

2–5 years age group

Arises from kidney

Relatively well-defined, homogenous tumor associated with areas of hemorrhage and necrosis, leading to distortion of renal architecture and displacement of collecting system

NEUROBLASTOMA

Second most common abdominal tumor of childhood

2 months—2 years

Arises from the adrenal gland or sympathetic chain (extrarenal)

Relatively poorly defined, heterogeneous tumor with calcifications, displacing and compressing the kidney without distortion of renal architecture

Encases vascular structures but does not invade them

Elevates aorta away from the vertebral column

Commonly crosses the midline

Spreads early and widely with majority of patients presenting with metastasis

MESOBLASTIC NEPHROMA (FETAL RENAL HAMARTOMA, AND CONGENITAL WILM'S TUMOR)

Most common neonatal neoplasm to occur in the first few months of life.

Benign, but spreads with local invasion.

Solid neoplasm within kidney with areas of hemorrhage and necrosis.

RHABDOMYOSARCOMA (SARCOMA BOTRYOIDES)

Involves bladder base

Cluster of grapes appearance (anechoic spaces due to necrosis and hemorrhage)

Common in males

Presents as bladder outlet obstruction

Adrenals Glands

8

INTRODUCTION

Smallest paired organ in suprarenal location in the abdomen.

Weighs ~4 grams each in the normal nonstressed adult.

Though CT is a better imaging modality, USG may be helpful depending on the operator experience, patient's body habitus, and type of equipment.

In the neonatal period, normal adrenal gland can be visualized readily because of its relatively large size and little perirenal fat.

V/Y/Z shaped.

Long linear structure lying flat (*Lying down sign* in patients with renal agenesis).

PATHOLOGIES

Infectious diseases

Tuberculosis and histoplasmosis—Bilateral, diffuse enlargement, heterogeneous echotexture with calcifications.

HIV+ patient's demonstrate heterogeneously hypoechoic masses, may contain gas.

Adrenal abscess—common in neonates.

Neoplastic lesion

ADENOMAS

On USG

- Solid, small, round well-defined lesions in suprarenal region (Figure 8.1)

- In a parasagittal plane, if RUQ retroperitoneal fat stripe is displaced
  Posteriorly: It is s/o hepatic and subhepatic masses.
  Anteriorly: It is s/o kidney and adrenal masses.

CT and MRI scan should be recommended for further evaluation.

MYELOLIPOMAS

Incidental detection.

On USG, visualized as an echogenic mass in the suprarenal region.

If small, it is difficult to differentiate from the adjacent echogenic retroperitoneal fat.

CT scan is sensitive to detect fat containing lesions.

PHEOCHROMOCYTOMAS

Excessive secretion of catecholamines resulting in episodes of hypertension, severe headache, palpitations, and excessive sweating.

Only 10% are bilateral, malignant, extraadrenal, familial, found in children, not associated with hypertension, and contain calcification.

Measure the level of 24 hours urinary catecholamines, vanillylmandelic acid (VMA), and total metanephrines.

On USG, large homo/heterogeneous masses with areas of hemorrhage and necrosis.

I-131 MIBG scintigraphy is more sensitive.

Other benign neoplasms include ganglioneuromas, hemangiomas, and so on.

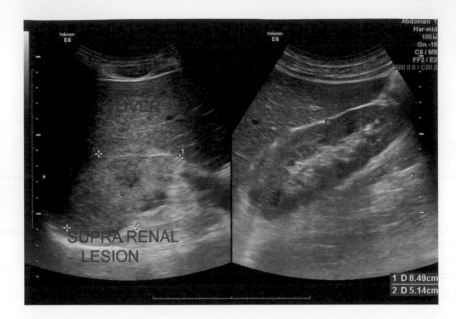

Figure 8.1 Well-defined heterogeneous lesion in the right suprarenal location.

ADRENAL METASTASES

Lymphoma: Discrete/conglomerate hypoechoic masses.

SARCOMAS

All are difficult to differentiate on USG.

Miscellaneous

ADRENAL CYSTS

Smooth-walled, well-defined anechoic cystic lesions.
Peripheral curvilinear calcifications may be seen in pseudocysts and parasitic adrenal cysts (echinococcal).

ADRENAL HEMORRHAGE

Associated with—Severe stress such as septicemia, burns, trauma, and hypotension.
In patients with hematological abnormalities.
Patients on anticoagulant therapy (within first 3 weeks of initiation of therapy).
Posttraumatic.
Seen usually on 2nd–7th day of life.
Presents as abdominal mass and hyperbilirubinemia.
Suprarenal mass with variable echogenicity (echogenic in acute stage and may become echo-free with clot liquefaction) on USG.
Usually occurs in the medulla of adrenal gland.
Resolves with time, usually requires no intervention.

WOLMAN'S DISEASE

Lipid storage disease.
Enlarged adrenal with diffuse punctuate calcifications.
Hepatosplenomegaly.

9

Aorta and Inferior Vena Cava

INTRODUCTION

Aorta enters the abdomen through the aortic
hiatus of the diaphragm, immediately anterior
to T-12 vertebra.

Descends anterior to and slightly to the left of
vertebral bodies.

Main branches seen on USG.

Celiac artery, superior mesenteric artery (SMA),
paired renal arteries, and common iliac arteries
(Figure 9.1).

Branches of aorta

1. Inferior phrenic artery
2. Celiac artery
3. Suprarenal artery
4. Superior mesenteric artery
5. Renal artery
6. Gonadal artery
7. Inferior mesenteric artery
8. Median sacral artery
9. Common iliac artery

Celiac artery demonstrates *seagull sign* and divides
into (Figure 9.2)

1. *Left gastric artery*: Supplies curvature of
   stomach
2. *Splenic artery*: Supplies greater curvature,
   spleen, and pancreas
3. *Common hepatic artery*: Divides into gastric
   artery, hepatic artery and gastroduodenal artery

Superior mesenteric artery supplies most of
the small intestine, ascending colon, and
part of the transverse colon.

Inferior mesenteric artery supplies part of
transverse colon, descending colon, and rectum.

Indications of USG

1. Pulsatile abdominal mass
2. Abdominal pain
3. Abdominal bruit
4. Hemodynamic compromise in lower limb arterial system

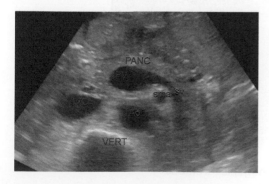

Figure 9.1 Depicting vascular anatomy after the
origin of SMA.

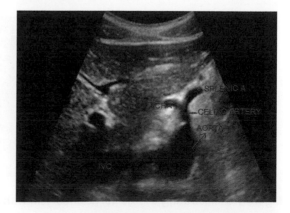

Figure 9.2 Illustrates origin and branching of
celiac artery *seagull sign*.

Normal aortic measurements

The abdominal aorta tapers from its cranial to its caudal extent and measures <2.3 centimeters in diameter for males and <1.9 centimeters for females. The upper limit varies with age and increased by up to 25%–30% in 70–80 years age group.

Atheromatous disease

Echogenic plaque causing mural irregularities and narrowing of vessel lumen.

Common in old age and men.

Associated with smoking, diabetes, hypertension, and dyslipidemia.

If significant lower limb pain is present, entire limb should be assessed by Doppler.

Circumferential narrowing of vessel lumen is also seen in Takayasu's arteritis.

Ectasia

Increase in both transverse diameter and vertical length of aorta causing a kink.

Aneurysm

Focal or generalized (>3 centimeters) dilatation of aorta (Figure 9.3).

True aneurysm: Lined by all three layers of aorta (intima, media, and adventitia).

False aneurysm: Pseudoaneurysm.

95% of aneurysms are infrarenal in location.

Complications include rupture, thrombosis, dissection, embolism, and infection.

Pseudoaneurysm

Breach in the vessel wall through which blood leaks and is contained by the adventitia. On Doppler, turbulent forward and backward flow is seen as *yin-yang* sign. *To and fro* pattern may be seen with pulsed Doppler.

Inferior vena cava

Large vein that returns blood from the lower limbs, pelvis, and abdomen to the right atrium.

Formed by the paired common iliac veins on the anterior surface of L-5 vertebra.

Main tributaries visualized on USG are hepatic veins, renal veins, and common iliac veins.

Gets mildly enlarged with right-sided heart failure and fluid overload.

Tributaries (from inferior to superior)

1. Common iliac veins
2. Lumbar veins
3. Right gonadal vein
4. Renal vein
5. Right suprarenal vein
6. Hepatic veins
7. Inferior phrenic vein

Left gonadal vein drains into the left renal vein.

Thrombosis: Echogenicity of a thrombus depends on its age. Color Doppler is helpful. In patients with HCC and RCC, IVC should be looked for thrombus.

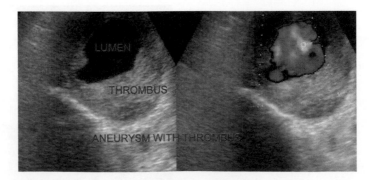

Figure 9.3 Illustrating a large aortic aneurysm with echogenic thrombus.

Leiomyosarcoma of the wall of IVC is the most common mural tumor in the venous system.

Ovarian vein thrombosis: Commonly seen in postpartum cases and is associated with endometritis and surgery. Enlarged ovarian vein with echogenic thrombus is seen on sonography. Usually occurs on the right side.

Points to note

IVC can be differentiated from aorta by

- IVC collapses during inspiration and expands during expiration.
- Flattened or oval cross section of IVC in comparison to aorta, which is round.
- IVC diameter is proportional to the right atrial pressure.
- IVC diameter reduces with inspiration.
  High intravascular volume show little change in IVC diameter with inspiration.
  Low intravascular volume show marked change and collapse of IVC with inspiration.

10

Pelvic USG (Uterus and Ovaries)

INTRODUCTION

Full bladder is required for pelvic USG as fluid in the urinary bladder facilitates transmission of sound waves for better visualization of uterus and ovaries.

Uterus

Prepubertal: Inverse pear shaped. Body of uterus is smaller than cervix.

Nonvisualized endometrial cavity.

Measures approximately

2 – 3.5 × 0.5 – 1.0 centimeters (L × AP).

Postpubertal: Nulliparous, pear shaped.

Measures approximately

4.5 – 9.0 × 1.5 – 3.0 × 4.5 – 5.5 centimeters (L × AP × T).

Uterine dimensions increase by 1–1.2 centimeters with parity and its body becomes rounded (Table 10.1).

Pattern of endometrium varies with menstrual cycle.

Anteroposterior diameter of cervix should not exceed that of uterine body.

Postmenopausal: Smaller and homogeneous with nonvisualization of endometrial cavity.

- Muscles in uterine walls appear hypoechoic.
- Posterior cul-de-sac (POD—Pouch of Douglas) is the most posterior and inferior reflection of peritoneal cavity located between rectum and vagina.
- Adnexa include ovaries, fallopian tubes, ligaments, and vessels.

Anteverted: Cervix and vagina forms a 90-degree angle (Figure 10.1).

Anteflexed: Body is flexed normally anteriorly on the cervix (270 degrees).

Retroverted: Uterus is tilted posteriorly toward the spine.

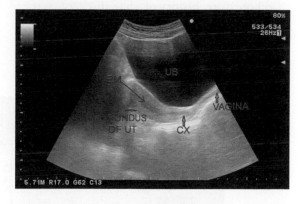

Figure 10.1 Showing normal echotexture of uterus, cervix, and vagina.

Table 10.1 Illustrates uterine dimensions in different stages of female

Uterus	Uterine length	Fundus: cervix	Endometrium
Newborn	3.5 centimeters	1:2	Bright endometrial stripe (due to *in utero* hormonal stimulation)
Prepubertal	2.5–3.5 centimeters	1:1	No endometrial stripe seen
Postpubertal	5–8 centimeters	3:1	Endometrium varies with menstrual phase

Leads to poor visualization of the endometrial cavity.

Visualization of broad ligament leads to widening of adnexa.

Fundus appears *echo poor* in appearance simulating a fundal fibroid.

No contour abnormality and displacement of endometrium differentiates it from fibroid. TVS is better.

Retroflexed: Fundus points backward. Cervix may be interposed between the probe and the body of uterus.

Cervix

Constricted lower part of the uterus connecting main body of the uterus to the vagina.

Nabothian cysts: Cysts within the cervix representing dilated or obstructed endocervical glands. Clinically not significant. Single cyst may sometimes simulate as low implanted gestational sac (Figure 10.2).

Bulky cervix: Anteroposterior diameter of cervix >~3.0 centimeters. Heterogeneous echotexture, history of white discharge warrants pap smear evaluation and follow-up.

May occur due to cervicitis, fibroid, and malignancy.

Vagina

Tubular structure with hypoechoic walls surrounding the central hyperechoic apposed surfaces of vaginal mucosa.

Ovaries

Bilateral oval, homogeneous structures lying laterally to the uterus with multiple well-defined anechoic follicles (Figure 10.3).

Ovarian volume—(L × W × AP) × 0.53 (Table 10.2).

Postmenopausal—1–6 cubic centimeters (>8 cubic centimeters is abnormal)—Ovaries are smaller, difficult to recognize. Sometimes they are hyperechoic without any follicles and similar to the surrounding tissues.

In some females up to 14–18 cubic centimeters of ovarian volume may be seen normally. Look for arrangement of follicles and stroma before diagnosing polycystic ovarian disease (PCOD) (Table 10.3).

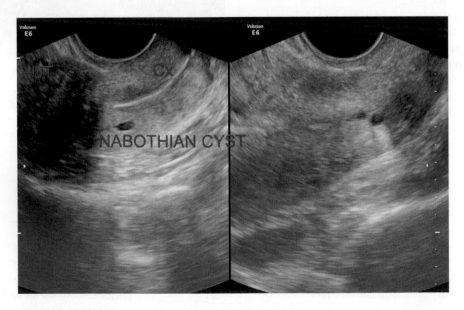

Figure 10.2 Showing multiple nabothian cysts in the cervix.

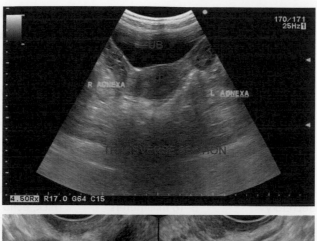

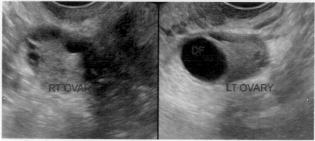

Figure 10.3 Depicting bilateral ovaries in the adnexa and a normal ovary showing multiple follicles with dominant follicle.

Table 10.2 Illustrating ovarian volume in different age groups of females

<5–6 years	<1 cc
6–11 years	1.0–2.5 cc
>11 years	up to 10 cc

Endometrium

Premenstrual: Hyperechogenic

Postmenstrual: Thin, hypoechoic line (Table 10.4 and Figure 10.4)

Postmenopausal (not on hormone replacement therapy [HRT]) <4 millimeters ideally or maximum 8 millimeters

Table 10.3 Illustrating varying appearances of ovary in different stages of menstrual cycle

Days of menstrual cycle	Appearance
5–7 days	Multiple small anechoic follicles in the ovary.
8–12 days	One dominant follicle can be recognized, which increases in size up to 16–28 millimeters.
24 hours before ovulation	Cumulus oophorus may be seen.
At the time of ovulation	Follicle ruptures, expels the ovum into fallopian tubes. The remnants of the follicle are known as corpus luteum, which produces estrogen and progesterone for sustaining favorable conditions for implantation of ovum, if it gets fertilized. Follicle reduces in size and may be filled with echogenic debris. May retain fluid over next 4–5 days and increases in size to 2–5 centimeters. *Corpus haemorrhagicum*—if bleeding occurs into the follicle. *Corpus albicans*—if no pregnancy occurs and corpus luteum involutes.

Table 10.4 Illustrating appearance of endometrium during different phases of the menstrual cycle

Date of cycle	Phase	Thickness	Appearance
1–4 days	Menstrual	1–4 millimeters	Thin interrupted central echo Small amount of fluid seen endovaginally
5–14 days	Proliferative	4–8 millimeters	Central echogenic line surrounded by thin hypoechoic (dark) band
	Periovulatory	6–10 millimeters	Trilayered appearance Dark band with thin echogenic line on either side
15–28 days	Secretory	8–16 millimeters	Thick, echogenic endometrium

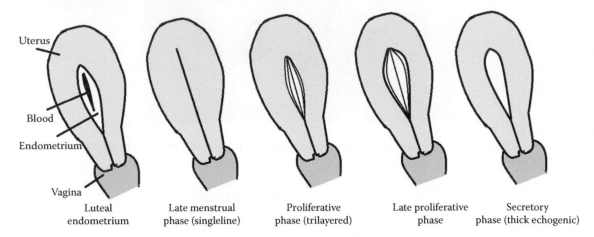

Figure 10.4 Illustrating varying appearances of endometrium depending on phases of menstrual cycle.

On HRT

Sequential HRT: Monthly withdrawal bleeding and cyclical endometrial thickening. At mid cycle 8–15 millimeters.

Continuous HRT: No cyclical endometrial changes with maximum 8 millimeters thickness.

ABNORMAL UTERINE BLEEDING

Etiology

1. Exclude pregnancy by urinary pregnancy test (UPT)
2. Dysfunctional/anovulatory uterine bleeding (DUB) is the most common cause (termed as hormonal imbalance)
3. Organic pathologies—Submucous myomas, polyps, hyperplasia, and carcinoma

Endometrial pathology

In postmenopausal patients

- Thin, distinct endometrial echo <4–5 millimeters—high negative predictive value.
- Endometrial fluid collection with thin endometrium surrounding the fluid s/o inactive atrophic endometrium (secondary to cervical stenosis).
- Endometrial fluid collection—Endometrial tissue surrounding the fluid is thick and irregular suggestive of endometrial hyperplasia with atypia. Suggest saline infusion sonohysterogram.
- Polyp—Look for a feeder vessel.
- Submucous fibroid.

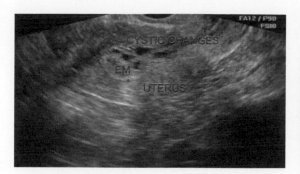

Figure 10.5 Illustrating thickened endometrium with cystic changes on a patient with carcinoma breast on tamoxifen.

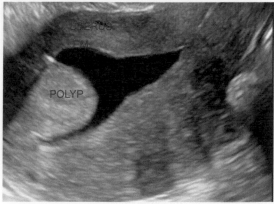

Figure 10.6 Illustrating endometrium polyp in saline hysterography.

K/C/O carcinoma breast on tamoxifen—Microcystic changes due to glandular cystic atrophy (Figure 10.5).

Endometrial polyps

Localized overgrowth of endometrial glands and stroma can be

- Sessile
- Pedunculated

Three types:

Hyperplastic: Resembles glands of endometrial hyperplasia.
Atrophic: Cystic and dilated atrophic glands.
Functional: Undergo cyclical endometrial change.
Feeder vessel (Pedicle) seen entering the endometrium.
Common in perimenopausal and postmenopausal females.
USG—Endocavitary iso/hyperechoic mass surrounded by fluid (Figure 10.6).
D/D submucous fibroid—Broad base and irregular contour.
  Normal layer of overlying endometrium can be appreciated.
Sonohysterography is diagnostic, in which 5 milliliters saline is infused into the endometrial cavity through a catheter during TVS.

Endometrial hyperplasia

Excessive proliferation of endometrial glands.
  Thickening is hypovascular to differentiate from hypervascular carcinoma (Figure 10.7).
Due to unopposed estrogen stimulation (anovulatory, states, obesity, tamoxifen therapy).
S/s—Postmenopausal bleeding.
  Simple: Cystic → cystic dilation of glands with abundant cellular stroma.
  Complex: Adenomatous—More number of glands with scanty stroma.
In symptomatic postmenopausal female, endometrium >5 millimeters → abnormal
In asymptomatic postmenopausal female, endometrium >5–8 millimeters → abnormal

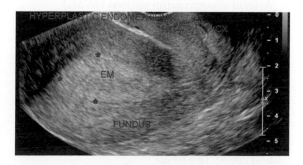

Figure 10.7 Illustrating thickened hyperplastic endometrium.

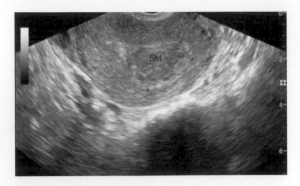

Figure 10.8 Illustrating thickened, heterogeneous endometrium.

In premenopausal, it is abnormal if
In proliferative phase >8 millimeters
In secretory phase >16 millimeters

Endometrial synechiae/adhesions: Asherman's—Due to trauma, infection, and inflammation.

Irregular, hypoechoic, and bridge-like bands within the endometrium (best seen in the secretory phase).

Endometrial carcinoma

Irregularly thickened endometrium with increased vascularity and indistinct interface with myometrium in a postmenopausal female with vaginal bleeding, suggesting the importance of clinical history and age of the patient (Figure 10.8).

Biopsy is confirmatory.

MENORRHAGIA

Causes

1. Fibroids
2. Adenomyosis
3. Arterio venous malformations (AVMs)
4. Postpartum/Post dilatation & curettage (D&C)
5. IUCD

Fibroids (Leiomyomas)

Most common gynecological disorder of the reproductive age group.

Usually benign, of myometrial origin and consists of predominantly smooth muscle with fibrous and connective tissue.

Estrogen dependent. Frequently increases in size during pregnancy and diminishes after menopause.

SIGNS AND SYMPTOMS

Can be asymptomatic. May present with pain, abnormal bleeding (menorrhagia), and pressure effects on adjacent pelvic organs.

USG

1. Enlarged uterus with distortion of uterine contour.
2. Well circumscribed with pseudocapsule.
3. Variegated pattern of echogenicity.
4. May be multiple.
5. Hyaline, cystic, myxoid, and calcific degeneration may occur due to lack of blood supply.

TYPES

1. *Intramural*: Most common, seen in the anterior/posterior myometrium (Figure 10.9).
2. *Submucosal*: Broad-based hypoechoic masses with an overlying layer of echogenic endometrium causing distortion of endometrial complex. Most important D/D is endometrial polyp, which shows feeding vessel on color Doppler.
3. *Subserosal*: Pedunculated, mainly extrauterine, simulates adnexal lesion, and may exert pressure on adjacent organs, if large in size.

Red/Carneous degeneration may occur—Patient presents with acute abdominal pain due to hemorrhagic infarction mostly seen during pregnancy. Unusual signal intensity patterns are diagnosed on MRI.

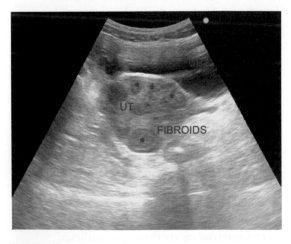

Figure 10.9 Illustrating multiple small intramural fibroids.

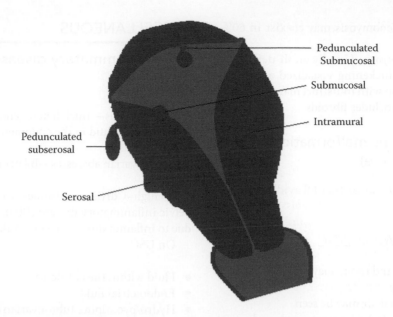

Figure 10.10 Demonstrating various patterns of fibroids.

OTHER D/Ds

Lipomas/Lipoleiomyoma—Centrally hyperechoic with a hypoechoic rim
Focal myometrial contractions during pregnancy
Focal adenomyosis
Teratomas
Sarcomas (malignant) (Figure 10.10)

BROAD LIGAMENT FIBROID

May present as pelvic pain and pressure on adjacent organs.

Extrauterine leiomyoma, it is seen as solid, hypoechoic (or heterogeneous), well-circumscribed adnexal mass separated from both the uterus and ovary. Torsion may occur, if it is pedunculated.

D/Ds—Solid adnexal neoplasms, subserosal leiomyoma projecting toward broad ligament.

Sometimes a pedunculated subserosal fibroid outgrows its blood supply from the uterus and acquires new blood supply from the structures adherent to it such as the omentum. It is known as *parasitic leiomyoma* and should be considered in differentials of adnexal lesion when uterus and ovary are seen separately.

DIFFUSE LEIOMYOMATOSIS

Rare entity, involves diffuse involvement of myometrium by innumerable small fibroids leading to symmetrical enlargement of uterus.

Seedling fibroids: Sometimes tiny fibroids, not altering the contour of uterus are present, best visualized on TVS. May be asymptomatic or may present with menorrhagia.

Adenomyosis

Defined as ectopic endometrial tissue in the myometrium.
Common in mature reproductive age group than nulliparous and postmenopausal females.
S/S—uterine tenderness, dysmenorrhea, menorrhagia.

TRANSABDOMINAL SONOGRAPHY

Enlarged globular uterus without focal masses, mostly involving posterior myometrium.

TRANSVAGINAL SONOGRAPHY

- Heterogeneously hypoechoic posterior myometrial echotexture with hyperechoic foci.
- Shaggy endometrium with poor differentiation between the endometrium and the myometrium.
- Asymmetrical thickened myometrium.
- Tiny subendometrial and myometrial cysts <5 millimeters.
- Smooth external contour.
- Lack of calcifications and mass effect on serosa or endometrium.

Fibroids and adenomyosis may coexist in 60% of patients.

Focal adenomyosis: Usually an ill-defined area of myometrial thickening visualized as heterogeneous focal lesion with indistinct margins and cystic spaces. D/D includes fibroids.

Arterio venous malformations (Vascular tangle)

Serpigenous cystic areas that fill avidly with color on Doppler.

Postpartum/post D&C

<3 days—Fluid and tissue may be seen in the uterine cavity.
~7 days—Residual air may be seen.
If bleeding persists, look for retained products of conception (RPOC).
Gravid uterus diminishes in size with rapid decrease in—1–2 weeks and returns to normal by 6–8 weeks.

Postpartum USG done for

1. Retained products of conception—Heterogeneous echogenic lesion with vascularity seen in the endometrium after delivery, D&C, and medical abortion (Figure 10.11).
2. Continuous bleeding, pain, and vaginal discharge after delivery.

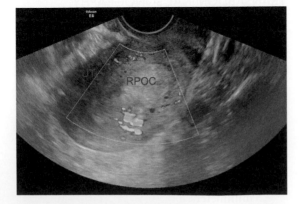

Figure 10.11 Illustrating RPOC after D&C.

MISCELLANEOUS

Pelvic inflammatory disease

Stages

1. Endometritis—Thick heterogenous endometrium with fluid in the endometrial canal.
2. Salpingitis.
3. Tubo-ovarian abscesses—Bilateral pyosalpinx.

Fitz–Hugh–Curtis syndrome—Complication of pelvic inflammatory disease (PID); a/w RUQ pain due to inflammation of liver capsule.
On USG

- Fluid within the cul-de-sac
- Endometrial fluid
- Hydro/pyosalpinx tubo-ovarian abscess (TOA) (Figure 10.12)
- Mild uterine enlargement

Arcuate artery calcification

Normal arcuate vessels are seen as hypoechoic tubular structures with color flow on the Doppler.
Calcification is noticed as asymmetric, echogenic foci with acoustic shadowing in the periphery of myometrium of the uterus.
Seen in patients with diabetes, atherosclerosis, hypertension, and chronic renal failure.

Pelvic congestion syndrome

Presentation: Chronic noncyclical pain, worsening with standing, sitting, and during menses

- Dyspareunia
- Generalized weakness, abdominal tenderness
- Bladder and bowel discomfort
- Hemorrhoids and varices

USG: Dilated ovarian veins >4 millimeters

Dilated, tortuous arcuate myometrial veins
May extend to pelvis

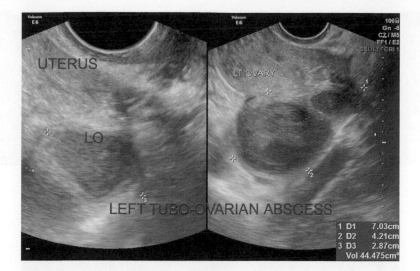

Figure 10.12 Illustrating left tubo-ovarian abscess with echogenic debris.

Hematometrocolpos

Distension of uterus, cervix, and vagina (colpos) with blood (nonpassage of menstrual blood) secondary to obstruction/atresia of lower reproductive tract (cervix/vagina).

ETIOLOGY

Congenital: Imperforate hymen, transverse vaginal septum, and hypoplastic vagina
Aquired: Cervical stenosis, intrauterine adhesions carcinoma of endometrium and cervix

D/D Pyometra: Uterus filled with pus

Vaginal cysts

Gartner duct cyst: Located in the anterolateral wall of vagina proximally. Lies at or above the level of pubic symphysis.
Bartholin's cyst: Commonly unilocular, lies at the posterior part of the vagina at or below the level of pubic symphysis. May develop into abscess if gets infected.

CYSTIC MASSES OF PELVIS

1. Physiological—Follicular, corpus luteal cysts
2. Hemorrhagic cysts
3. Simple ovarian cysts
4. Polycystic ovarian disease (PCOD)
5. Hydrosalpinx
6. Cystadenoma (Serous/Mucinous)
7. Parovarian cysts
8. Peritoneal inclusion cysts
9. Endometrioma
10. Theca lutein cysts

Follicular cysts/functional cysts

Develops when a follicle fails to ovulate
Usually in females of reproductive age group
Unilocular, anechoic cyst with thin wall with posterior acoustic enhancement (Figure 10.13a)
Approximately—3–5 centimeters in size
Spontaneous resolution seen
Follow-up usually in the first week of menstrual cycle and after 6 weeks is recommended

Corpus luteal cysts

Formed by the dominant follicle after ovulation. (Unilateral usually).
Follicle wall becomes vascularized, thickened, and partially collapsed (Luteinization).
Can cause periovulatory pain.
Prone to hemorrhage and rupture.
If the ovum gets fertilized → CL of pregnancy reaches maximum size at 8–10 weeks → resolves by 12–16 weeks.

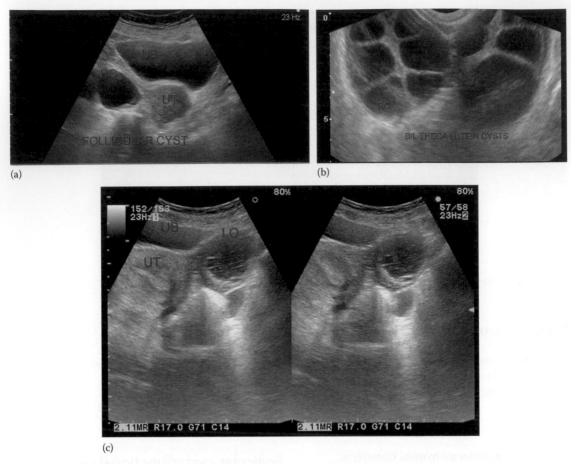

Figure 10.13 **(a)** Illustrating physiological follicular cyst, **(b)** illustrating bilateral theca lutein cysts, and **(c)** illustrating cyst with fine linear echoes.

On USG, appears as thick-walled cystic lesion with echogenic component (due to bleeding). *Ring of fire* appearance on color Doppler.

Theca lutein cysts (Figure 10.13b)

Multiple large cysts usually associated with high hCG levels (in gestational trophoblastic disease and patients on exogenous hCG for infertility).

Multilocular, bilateral large cysts.

May undergo hemorrhage, rupture, or torsion.

Hemorrhagic cysts (Figure 10.13c)

Cyst with fine linear echoes (fibrin strands), echogenic material, fluid–fluid level (fish-net appearance).

Retracting thrombus (with absence of blood flow) adherent to wall may be seen (D/D focal mural nodule).

Follow-up after 4–6 weeks, preferably in the first week of menstrual cycle is recommended.

Usually resolves on its own.

Polycystic ovarian disease (Stein–Leventhal syndrome)

Bilateral enlarged ovaries with multiple small anechoic follicles and thick echogenic stroma (string of pearls/necklace appearance) (Figure 10.14).

Presents with oligo/amenorrhea, hirsutism, obesity, or infertility.

High LH/FSH and androgen levels.

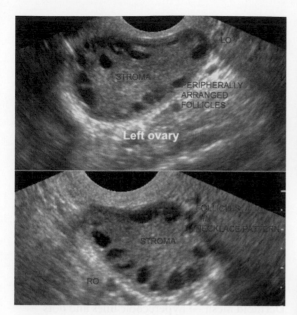

Figure 10.14 Illustrating multiple follicles arranged peripherally.

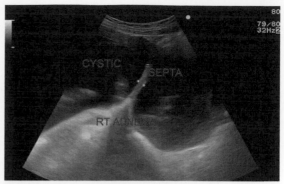

Figure 10.15 Demonstrates multiloculated septated cystic lesion in right adnexa.

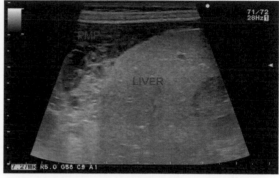

Figure 10.16 Illustrating pseudomyxoma peritonei after rupture of mucinous tumor.

Hydrosalpinx

Fluid-filled dilatation of the fallopian tube due to its occlusion at the distal end.

Tubular, elongated extraovarian structure with incomplete septations, and folded configuration.

Absence of peristalsis to differentiate from the bowel. If it gets distended with pus or blood products (low-level echoes), it is called pyosalpinx or hematosalpinx, respectively.

Parovarian cysts

Anechoic cysts adjacent to and separate from the ovary.

Dimensions remain same throughout the menstrual cycle.

Usually seen in 30–40 years of age group.

Cystadenomas (Figure 10.15)

SEROUS CYSTADENOMAS

40–50 years.

Large (up to 10 centimeters), thin-walled unilocular cystic mass with thin septa and papillary projections.

MUCINOUS CYSTADENOMAS

30–50 years.

Large (up to 15–30 centimeters), multilocular with multiple septae, and low-level echoes.

Variegated echogenicity noted due to difference in chemical composition of fluids.

Papillary projections are less frequent.

Rupture may lead to intraperitoneal spread of mucin-secreting cells (pseudomyxoma peritonei) (Figure 10.16).

Tubo-ovarian abscess

Multilocular, complex thick-walled mass with irregular borders and internal septations.

Free fluid present.

Usually due to ascending infection involving endometrium and fallopian tube.

Follow-up is required to assess response to antibiotic therapy.

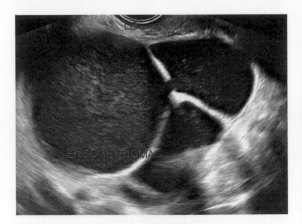

Figure 10.17 Illustrating cystic lesion with homogeneous low-level echoes.

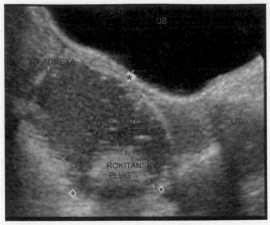

Figure 10.18 Illustrating complex cystic lesion with echogenic plug and fibrin strands.

Endometriosis (Figure 10.17)

Implantation of endometrium outside the uterus.

Most common sites—Ovary (80%), uterosacral ligaments, cul-de-sac, posterior wall of lower uterine segment, fallopian tube, rectovaginal septum, and sigmoid colon.

Bilateral in 30%–50% of cases.

Females of reproductive age group are affected mostly.

Presents with chronic lower abdominopelvic pain, backache, irregular bleeding, dysmenorrhea, infertility, and so on.

On USG, seen as well-defined cystic mass with homogeneous low-level echoes.

Repeated episodes of bleeding leads to development of irregular walls and echogenic mural nodules.

Fluid–fluid levels or fluid–debris levels represent blood products.

Hyperechoic wall foci, if seen, represent focal cholesterol deposits.

Dermoid/mature cystic teratomas (Figure 10.18)

Contains all the three germ layers.

Frequent in females of reproductive age group.

On USG, noted as complex cystic mass with solid mural component (dermoid plug).

May contain hair, teeth, or fat and is echogenic causing acoustic shadow.

High amplitude echoes within the mass are due to sebum.

Dermoid mesh → hyperechoic lines and dots within the mass.

Fat-fluid or hair-fluid level may be specific.

Peritoneal inclusion cysts

Usually seen in premenopausal females.

Associated with h/o trauma, abdominal surgery, endometriosis, and PID.

Normal peritoneum absorbs fluid produced by the ovaries.

Loss of the ability to absorb fluid (due to inflammation/ adhesions) → accumulation of fluid within the adhesions → entrapment of ovaries → large cystic, multiseptated adnexal mass with intact ovary lying centrally or in the wall of the cyst.

Ovarian torsion

Severe pain.

Free fluid.

Enlarged, edematous, and heterogeneous ovary with small cysts.

Venous blood flow is compromised followed by arterial compromise in severe cases only because of dual blood supply to ovary.

MISCELLANEOUS

1. Bowel within the pelvis sometimes simulates as a cystic lesion. Review scan after few minutes or hours will resolve the issue.

2. Streak ovaries—Small stripe of fibrous tissue without follicles noted in the anticipated location of ovaries. May be visualized in Turner's syndrome (XO, gonadal dysgenesis).

MALIGNANT LESIONS OF PELVIS

Carcinoma endometrium

Risk factors: Prolonged estrogen stimulation (oral contraceptive pills [OCPs], postmenopausal HRT, tamoxifen therapy), nulliparity, obesity, and diabetes.

Age group: >50 years.

Presentation: Postmenopausal bleeding, discharge.

USG

Thickened endometrium.

>5 millimeters in postmenopausal females (up to 7 millimeters in women on estrogen therapy).

>15 millimeters in symptomatic premenopausal females.

Irregularity of endomyometrial invasion is s/o invasion.

If tumor is large, it enlarges and distorts uterine echotexture.

Look for lymphadenopathy, involvement of cervix and vagina, and parametrial involvement.

Carcinoma cervix (Mostly squamous cell carcinoma)

Risk factors: Early age at first coitus

Multiple sexual partners

Sexually transmitted human papilloma virus (HPV) infection

Presentation: Foul smelling white discharge, vaginal bleeding, and pelvic pain.

USG

- An ill-defined, heterogeneously isoechoic (not easily identifiable) lesion leading to bulky cervix (Figure 10.19).
- When large and necrotic, tumors are hypoechoic, easily identifiable.
- Presence of hydro/pyometra is s/o endocervical canal obstruction.
- May involve vagina, parametrium, bladder, and rectum.
- May cause iliac and retroperitoneal lymphadenopathy and distant metastasis.
- May cause hydronephrosis. Kidneys should always be scanned in carcinoma cervix.

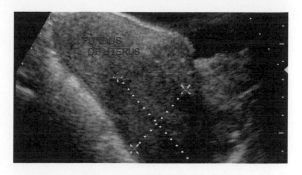

Figure 10.19 Illustrating heterogeneously enlarged cervix, later proved as carcinoma.

Post radiotherapy: Tumor and uterus reduces in size. Edema/necrosis may mimic residual tumor. Follow-up USG and Pap (Papanikolaou) smear for minimum 5 years.

Recurrence: Vaginal vault and lymph nodes are the common sites for recurrence.

CT/MRI scan for better characterization of the lesion.

Carcinoma vagina

Usually involves upper third of the vagina. Spreads to bladder and rectum along with pelvic lymphadenopathy.

Hematogenous metastasis.

Sarcoma of uterus

Associated with prior pelvic irradiation.

Areas of necrosis, hemorrhage, myometrial invasion, and peritoneal deposits seen.

Usually large at the time of presentation.

Rhabdomyosarcoma of uterus, cervix, and vagina—in children.

Clear cell adenocarcinoma of vagina—Associated with diethylstilbestrol (DES) exposure.

Multicystic expansile mass in vagina.

Ovarian tumors

Four types according to their cell of origin:

1. Epithelial—60%–70%
   Serous cystadenocarcinoma (B/L)
   Mucinous cystadenocarcinoma (U/L)
   Endometroid carcinoma (B/L)

Brenner's tumor (B/L)
Clear cell carcinoma (U/L)—better prognosis
2. Germ cell tumors (GCT)—15%–20%
Benign cystic teratomas—Dermoids
Malignant GCT's—Dysgerminomas
Immature teratoma (normal AFP and hCG)
Embryonal tumor (high AFP and hCG)
Yolk sac tumor (High AFP)—Rapid growth,
early metastasis
Choriocarcinoma (high hCG)
3. Sex cord stromal tumors—5%–10%
Fibromas
Thecomas
Arrhenoblastomas (Sertoli cell/Leydig cell
tumors)
Granulosa cell tumors
4. Metastasis

Malignant ovarian tumors

80% occur in females >50 years

Presentation: Pain, abdominal distension,
vaginal bleeding, bladder, and bowel
dysfunction
Risk factors: Family history of cancers, BRCA 1/2
genetic mutation
Nulliparous
Treatment with ovulation-induction agents
Protection: Multiparity, breast feeding, use of
OCPs

Features s/o benign pathology

Size <5 centimeters, thin wall, and thin septations
Absence of color flow
High resistive index

Features s/o malignancy (Figure 10.20)

Heterogeneous hypoechoic, complex cystic lesion
Thick irregular walls
Thick (>3 millimeters) nodular septations
Size >7 centimeters with a solid mural nodule or
papillary projections
Poorly defined margins

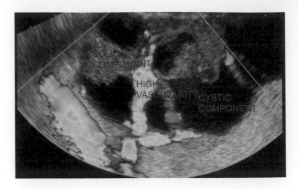

Figure 10.20 Illustrating septated cystic lesion with a solid component and increased vascularity.

Adherent bowel loops
Ascites
Peritoneal nodules and omental thickening s/o
metastasis
Lymphadenopathy
On Doppler
Central vascularity
High impedance flow with RI <0.4

Serous cystadenocarcinoma—60%–80% cases.

Cystic, septated lesion with internal solid areas
and wall thickening.
60%–70% are bilateral.

Mucinous cystadenocarcinoma

Cystic mass, multiloculated with thick septations,
and internal echoes due to high mucin content
(Variegated echogenicity sign—variable
echogenicities in different locules).
May be associated with septated ascites and
lymphadenopathy.
Pseudomyxoma peritonei due to intraperitoneal
spread of mucin cells leading to gelatinous
deposits throughout the peritoneum and
scalloping of liver, spleen, and bowel surface.
5%–10% are bilateral.

Endometroid carcinoma

Usually associated with endometrial hyperplasia
and endometriosis.

Malignant germ cell tumors

Seen in young females (~20–30 years)
U/L, solid, well defined with cystic/necrotic/
hemorrhagic areas
Large solid tumors associated with high levels of
hCG, AFP, and CA-125

Metastasis (Krukenberg's tumor)

Common primary sites—Stomach, colon, and
breast.
Krukenberg tumor—Histological pattern of
mucin secreting signet cells with sarcomatous
stroma usually from gastric primary.
Bilateral, large, lobulated, and complex solid—
Cystic lesions associated with ascites, peritoneal nodules, and omental deposits.

Meig's syndrome

Triad of
Fibromas (ovarian)
Slow-growing ascites
Benign pleural effusion

Sex cord stromal tumors

Estrogen producing.
Presents with sexual precocity in prepubertal girls
and resumption of menses in postmenopausal
females.

Borderline malignant tumors have better
prognosis, low risk of local recurrence, and
metastasis.

CLASSIFICATION

Benign tumors

CYSTIC

Serous cystadenoma
Mucinous cystadenoma
Dermoid

SOLID

Brenner's tumor
Thecomas
Fibromas
Sertoli cell tumor

Malignant tumors

CYSTIC

Serous cystadenocarcinoma
Mucinous cystadenocarcinoma
Endometroid carcinoma

SOLID

Dysgerminomas—most common
Endodermal sinus tumor (yolk sac tumor)
Endometroid granulosa cell tumor
Metastasis

11

Prostate

INTRODUCTION

A gram of prostate tissue is equivalent to 1 milliliter of volume; hence, volume could be converted to weight.

Prostate: Chestnut shaped, homogeneous, and hypoechoic gland with <5 milliliters in size up to 12 years.

Seminal vesicles: Paired, hypoechoic structures cephalad to the base of the prostate; usually ~1 centimeter front to back.

Zonal anatomy

Four glandular zones surround the prostatic urethra:

1. Peripheral zone (PZ)—70% site for most prostatic cancers.
2. Transitional zone (TZ)—5% site of origin of benign prostatic hyperplasia (BPH).
3. Central zone (CZ)—25% relatively resistant to disease process. Only 5% cancers start here.
4. Periurethral area—1% internal prostatic sphincter.

On USG, it is difficult to identify these zones in normal prostate and only two zones are identified.

Outer gland: Peripheral (PZ + CZ)
Inner gland: (TZ + anterior fibromuscular stroma + internal urethral sphincter)

Both outer and inner glands are separated by a surgical capsule.

Neurovascular bundle lies bilaterally along the posterolateral aspect of the prostate and is a preferential pathway of tumor spread.

Corpora amylacea, seen as echogenic foci, develop along the surgical capsule and periurethral glands (proteinaceous debris in dilated prostatic ducts).

Measurements (Figure 11.1)

Maximal transverse width (*T*): Right to left
Anteroposterior (AP): Anterior midline to rectal surface
Length (*L*): Maximal head to foot

Volume is calculated by the formula

$$V = 1.57(T * AP * L)$$

Repeat-ability of volume measurements is not perfect and is within ±10%.

Normal prostate has volume of approximately 25 milliliters.

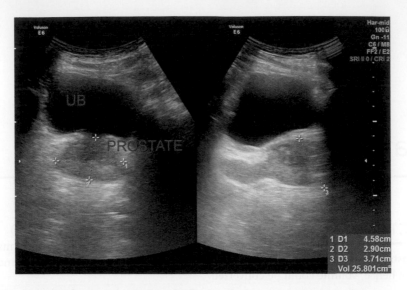

Figure 11.1 Depicting prostatic measurements in AP and transverse planes.

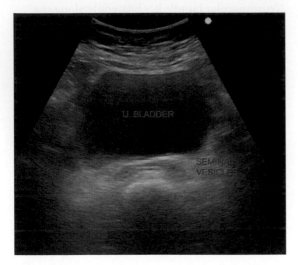

Figure 11.2 Illustrating normal paired seminal vesicles.

Seminal vesicles (Figure 11.2)

Paired accessory sex glands of male reproductive system, located posterosuperior to the prostate.
It may get inflamed causing heterogeneous echotexture due to seminal vesiculitis.

Transrectal ultrasonography

Better as it has ability to visualize the prostate in real time.

Benign ductal ectasia

Normal variant with no clinical significance.
Atrophy and dilatation of peripheral prostatic ducts. Radially oriented hypoechoic ducts. Unwary practitioners may mistake for prostate cancer.

Benign prostatic hyperplasia

In young patients, the prostate weighs <20 grams.
In older men, >25–30 grams is considered enlarged depending on symptoms.

On USG:

- Enlarged gland with inhomogeneous echotexture with nodularity (Figure 11.3)
- Degenerative cysts may be seen
- Increased postvoid residual volume
- Bladder wall trabeculation, diverticulae
- Prominent/enlarged median lobe indenting/protruding into the bladder

Patients who have transurethral resection of prostate (TURP) initially have funnel-shaped defect, which decreases in size as the gland collapses into the defect.

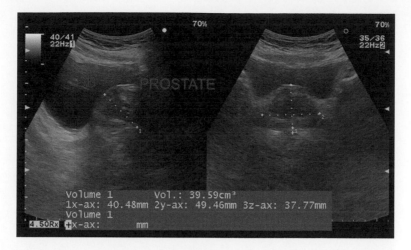

Figure 11.3 Illustrating measurements in benign hyperplasia of prostate.

Prostatitis

May be associated with chlamydia or
mycoplasma.
USG may be normal. May show-
Geographical (focal) masses of different degrees of
echogenicity.
Capsular thickening and irregularity.
Ejaculatory duct calcifications.
Distended seminal vesicles.
Dilated periprostatic veins with increased vascularity.
May mimic cancer and is associated with elevated
PSA.
Abscess—cystic anechoic area with echoes are s/o
abscess.
May be associated with cystitis and pain while
defecation.

Cysts

1. Degenerative or retention cysts may be seen; no
clinical significance.
2. Prostatic utricle cyst—Midline due to dilated
prostatic utricle. May be associated with
unilateral renal agenesis.
3. Seminal vesicles cysts—If solitary and large
associated with ipsilateral renal agenesis.

Prostate cancer

70% arise in PZ, 20% in TZ, and 10% in CZ.
Usually multifocal.

Cancers in PZ and CZ are usually homogeneous
and iso/hypoechoic.
Cancers in TZ are heterogeneous.
On USG, hypo/hyper/isoechoic nodules may
be seen.

Staging

T1—Confined to prostate; clinically not
palpable.
T2—Confined to prostate; clinically palpable.
T3—Extend through the prostatic capsule. May
involve seminal vesicles.
T4—Invades adjacent structures such as bladder,
rectum, and levator muscles.

PSA levels

<4 nanogram per milliliter—Normal
4–10 nanogram per milliliter—Indeterminate
>10 nanogram per milliliter—Abnormal
PSA more than 10 times the normal is highly suggestive of cancer.
Low PSA levels are noted with seen with finaste-
ride, saw palmetto and herbal medications.

TRUS is better for screening, cancer detection,
biopsy guidance, staging, therapy guidance, and
monitoring response to treatment. However, it is
not used for detecting extracapsular spread. MRI
is better.

Figure 3.3 illustrating measurements in benign hyperplasia of prostate

Prostatitis

May be associated with chlamydia or mycoplasma.

USG may be normal. May show—

Cytostrophic (focal) masses of differing degrees of echogenicity.

Capsule thickening and penetration.

Ejaculatory duct calcification.

Obstructed seminal vesicles.

Dilated periprostatic veins with increased vascularity.

May indicate cancer and is associated with elevated PSA.

Abscess—cystic anechoic area with echoes suggesting abscesses.

May be associated with pyuria and pain while delivery.

Cysts

1. Discreate with smooth margins and features, seen no effect of nodule.

2. Posterior midline cysts—utricle, Müllerian duct, etc. May be associated with infertility, etc.

3. Seminal vesicle cysts—solitary with large, associated with ipsilateral renal agenesis.

Prostate cancer

70% arise in PZ, 20% in TZ and 10% in CZ, usually multifocal.

Cancers in PZ and CZ are usually homogeneous and isoechoic.

Cancers in TZ are heterogeneous.

On USG, hypoechoic/isoechoic nodules may be seen.

Staging

T1—Confined to prostate, clinically not palpable.

T2—Confined to prostate, clinically palpable.

T3—Extend through the prostatic capsule, slay into other seminal vesicles.

T4—Involve adjacent structures such as bladder, rectum, and levator muscles.

PSA value

Prostate-specific antigen—usual 4–10 nanogram per ml, then. . . .

[10 nanogram per ml then multitude there have . . . .

PSA more than 30 times the normal is highly suggestive of cancer.

Low PSA levels are noted with seen with metastatic prostatitis and benign conditions.

TRUS is better for screening, cancer detection, biopsy guidance, staging, therapy guidance, and monitoring response to treatment. However, it is not used for detecting extracapsular spread. MRI is better.

Peritoneum and Retroperitoneum

12

INTRODUCTION

List of retroperitoneal organs

1. Kidneys, ureters
2. Uterus, fallopian tubes, prostate
3. Pancreas
4. Aorta, IVC
5. Esophagus (thoracic), duodenum (Second, third, and fourth)
6. Ascending and descending colon, rectum (middle one-third)
7. Adrenal glands

List of intraperitoneal organs

1. Liver, spleen
2. Stomach, duodenum (first part)
3. Jejunum, ileum
4. Cecum, appendix

5. Transverse and sigmoid colon, rectum (upper one-third)
6. Ovaries

Urinary bladder, lower one-third rectum, and distal ureters are infra/subperitoneal in nature.

Peritoneal cavity spaces

Small bowel mesentery is a specialized peritoneal fold extending from the second lumbar vertebra to the right iliac fossa containing blood vessels, nerves, lymph nodes, and fat. It connects jejunum and ileum to posterior abdominal wall and is difficult to appreciate if ascites is not present (Table 12.1).

Omentum: Specialized peritoneal folds.
Lesser omentum: Connects the lesser curvature of the stomach and proximal duodenum with the liver.

Table 12.1 Illustrating various peritoneal cavity spaces

Subphrenic space	Bilateral, inferior to diaphragm
Subhepatic space	Inferior to liver; anterior and posterior
	Posterior subhepatic space is called Morrison's space
Lesser sac (Omental bursa)	Between stomach and pancreas
Paracolic gutters	Bilateral; along ascending and descending colon.
	Right paracolic gutter is larger than left, communicates freely with the right subphrenic space
	Phrenicocolic ligament partially limits the connection between left paracolic gutter and left subphrenic space
Pelvic	Females—b/w uterus and rectum; also known as rectouterine pouch or POD (Pouch of Douglas)
	Males—recto vesical pouch; b/w rectum and urinary bladder
Anterior cul-de-sac	Urinary bladder and uterus

Greater omentum: Descends from the greater curvature of the stomach.

Foramen of Winslow (Epiploic foramen): Passage between greater and lesser sac.

Retroperitoneal spaces

1. Posterior pararenal space
2. Anterior pararenal space
3. Perirenal space

Ascites (Figure 12.1)

Normally, 50–75 milliliters of free fluid is present in the peritoneal cavity, acting as lubricant.

Excessive accumulation of peritoneal fluid is called as ascites.

Can be classified as transudate or exudate depending on the protein content.

With the patient lying supine, free fluid tends to accumulate in five locations mainly the paracolic gutters (right and left), pelvis, perisplenic areas, and Morrison's pouch.

Ascites can be classified as minimal (fluid in one location), mild (two locations), moderate (three locations), marked (four locations), and massive (five locations).

Particulate Ascites: Free fluid with echoes suggesting the presence of blood, pus, or neoplastic cells in the fluid.

Hemoperitoneum: Seen in trauma, ruptured ectopic pregnancy, ruptured aneurysm, postsurgical, and patients on anticoagulants.

Chylous ascites: Lymph accumulates in the peritoneal cavity and seen as particulate ascites or a fluid level on USG because of layering of lymphatic fluid.

Visualized in lymphangioma, trauma, surgery, and so on.

Free fluid moves with change in the patient's position.

Loculated fluid has rounded margins, show mass effect with frequently displacing structures from their usual location. USG is superior to CT scan in the characterization of fluid.

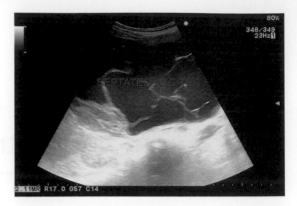

Figure 12.1 Depicting septated fluid collection in the peritoneal cavity.

Transvaginal USG can detect even 0.8 milliliter of free fluid.

Ascitic fluid volume estimation by sonography.

Width of fluid in Morrison's pouch (approximate values).

Small anechoic	stripe—250 milliliters
0.5 centimeter	stripe—500 milliliters
1.0 centimeter	stripe—1.0 liter

Retroperitoneum pathologies

LYMPHADENOPATHY

Round to oval hypoechoic lesion with poor sound transmission and absence of echogenic hilum (Figure 12.2).

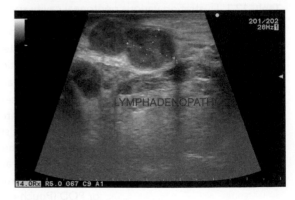

Figure 12.2 Illustrating lymphadenopathy.

Table 12.2 Illustrating criteria for evaluating nodal disease

Anatomic location	Size	Classification
Abdomen/ Pelvis	<1.0 centimeter	Normal
	>1.0 centimeter multiple	Abnormal
	>1.5 centimeter single	Abnormal
Retrocrural	>0.6 centimeter	Abnormal

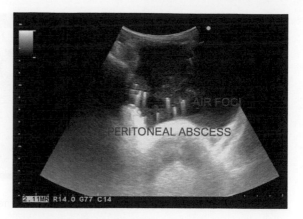

Figure 12.3 Demonstrating postoperative peritoneal abscess.

Most commonly due to lymphoma, infection, metastases (Germ cell tumors [GCT]; scrotum should be imaged in male patients), and so on (Table 12.2).

Sometimes, the nodes fuse to form hypoechoic mantle of tissue that surrounds the aorta and may elevate it from the spine.

Retroperitoneal fibrosis (Ormond's disease)

Idiopathic (68% cases)
Malignancy (infiltrating/secondaries)
Methysergide
Infection
Inflammatory aneurysms

Tumors

Primary retroperitoneal tumors: Usually mesenchymal in origin and include liposarcoma, leiomyosarcoma, and malignant fibrous histiocytoma. Teratomas may be seen in pediatric population.

Lymphoma and metastases

CT scan is better than USG.

Fluid collections (Figure 12.3)

Hematoma, abscesses, cysts, urinomas, lymphoceles (postsurgery), and lymphangioma.

MISCELLANEOUS

Horseshoe kidney, loop of aperistaltic bowel, and low-lying pancreas sometimes simulates a mass.

Psoas abscess: Hypoechoic, irregular thick-walled collection with internal echoes seen in psoas muscle.

CT is the modality of choice for imaging retroperitoneum.

CYSTIC MASSES OF ABDOMEN

1. Mesenteric cysts
2. Peritoneal inclusion cysts
3. Lymphangiomas
4. Enteric duplication cysts
5. Dermoid cysts
6. Pseudocysts (infectious, inflammatory, or traumatic)

Mesenteric cysts

Vary in size from <1 centimeter to >25 centimeters filling the entire pelvic cavity.
May be simple or complex anechoic lesion with septations.

Peritoneal inclusion cysts

Normally, the fluid produced by active ovaries in premenopausal patients is absorbed by the peritoneum. This balance may get disturbed by

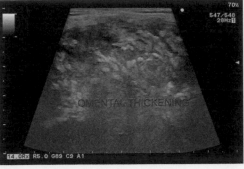 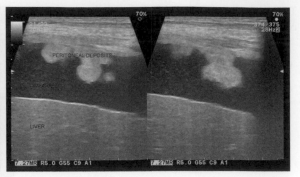

Figure 12.4 Illustrating peritoneal deposits and omental thickening.

surgery, trauma, or pathological processes. Fluid produced by ovaries gets trapped by adhesions. With time, an inclusion cyst forms that encases the normal varies and may cause pelvic pressure and pain.

D/d—ovarian cysts, hydrosalpinx.

Peritoneal tuberculosis

Loculated fluid collection with echoes and septations. Associated with mesenteric lymphadenopathy, bowel thickening, ascites, omental thickening, and peritoneal deposits (Figure 12.4).

Peritoneal carcinomatosis

Diffuse involvement of peritoneum with the metastatic disease.

On USG:

- Ascites.
- Hypoechoic nodules, irregular masses, or hypoechoic rind-like thickening of the peritoneum.
- Psammomatous calcifications, if present appear echogenic with posterior acoustic shadowing.
- Omental caking—Infiltration of omentum either adherent to peritoneum or floating freely in the ascites.
- Thickened mesentery, mesenteric nodules.
- Lymphadenopathy.

If the lesion remains stationary with respiration, parietal peritoneum involvement is suspected. If the lesion moves with respiration, visceral peritoneum involvement is suspected.

Primary peritoneal tumors—rare.
Malignant mesothelioma.
Lymphoma.

Chest

Chest USG can be done using suprasternal, parasternal, intercostal, subcostal, and subxiphoid approach; in supine, decubitus, and sitting position.

Pneumothorax is best visualized in anterior probe position.

Consolidation and effusions are best seen in posterior/lateral probe positions.

Two types of lines are seen:

A lines: Horizontal lines
B lines: Vertical lines
Interstitial lines with 7 millimeters spacing of interlobular septae.
Alveolar lines with 3 millimeters spacing of alveoli.

LUNG CONSOLIDATION (FIGURE 13.1)

Homogeneous, hypoechoic lung with echogenic punctate/linear branching structures (dynamic sonographic air bronchograms).

HEPATIZATION OF LUNG (FIGURE 13.2)

Echotexture of lung consolidation is similar to the liver in lobar pneumonia.

ATELECTASIS

Compressed, collapsed lung seen as wedge-shaped echogenic lung.

PLEURAL EFFUSION (FIGURES 13.3 AND 13.4)

USG can detect as little as—3–5 milliliters of fluid in the pleural cavity. It is usually echo-free and changes its shape with respiration. Transudates are usually sonolucent; exudates may contain floating echoes, fibrin strands, septations, s/o inflammatory, or neoplastic etiology.

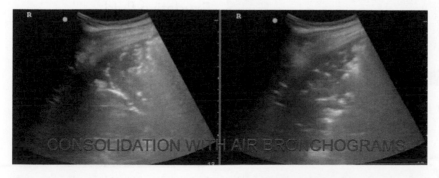

Figure 13.1 Illustrating lung consolidation with echogenic air bronchograms.

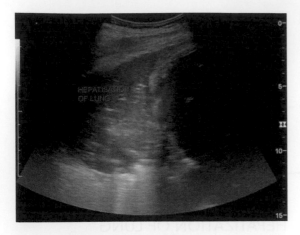

Figure 13.2 Illustrating hepatization of lung.

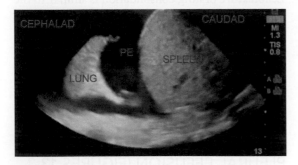

Figure 13.3 Demonstrates simple pleural effusion with collapsed lung.

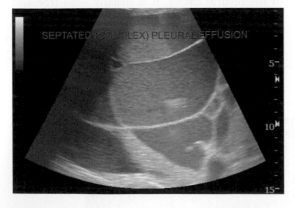

Figure 13.4 Illustrating complex pleural effusion.

On USG:

- Hypoechoic fluid collection under chest wall/above the diaphragm.
- Hyperechoic lung beneath fluid.

- Free fluid moves with respiration.
- *Diaphragm sign*: Pleural fluid is peripherally located and is outside the diaphragm in comparison to ascites, which is more centrally located and is inside the diaphragm.
- *Bare area sign*: Pleural fluid extends behind the liver at the level of the bare area in comparison to ascitic fluid, which cannot extend at the level of bare area.
- *Displaced crus sign*: Pleural fluid interposes between the crus and the vertebral column, displacing the crus away from the spine.

On color Doppler sonography (CDUS)—To differentiate between pleural effusion and thickening.

Color signal between the visceral and parietal pleura or near the costophrenic angle (related to respiratory movement) with chaotic to and fro turbulent flow-like signal is suggestive of pleural effusion.

Organized pleural thickening will appear as a colorless pleural lesion without any Doppler signal.

Transudative fluid

Congestive heart failure (CHF)
Cirrhosis
Glomerulonephritis
Nephrotic syndrome
Hypoalbuminemia
Overhydration

Exudative fluid

Infection
Neoplasm
Collagen vascular disease
Trauma
Drug induced

PNEUMOTHORAX

Lung-sliding sign: Normally, visceral and parietal pleural interfaces slide against one another due to presence of lubricating fluid in them known

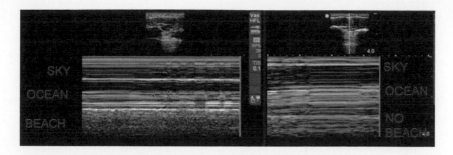

Figure 13.5 Illustrates *Sea Beach sign* with grainy pattern of normal lung and loss of grainy pattern (beach) in a patient with pneumothorax.

as lung sliding. However, this sign is absent in pneumothorax due to the presence of air in between the pleural layers.

However, this sliding may not be seen in cases with pleural adhesions or pleuritis.

Sea beach/stratosphere sign: Normally on M mode, pleural sliding will appear as grainy pattern (resembling sand of beach) beneath the chest wall—lung interface (resembles waves of sea at the beach as horizontal lines) (Figure 13.5).

However, in pneumothorax, grainy pattern is absent and is continued as horizontal lines.

DIAPHRAGM

Real-time sonography helps evaluate hemidia-phragms and their motion abnormalities.

Transducer is placed in a subxiphoid position with transverse orientation for bilateral and sagittal plane for unilateral hemidiaphragm.

Comparing maximal excursion of the diaphragm for each side.

Paralysis—Absent or paradoxical motion on one side and exaggerated excursions on the opposite side.

M mode helps in assessing diaphragmatic movement.

14

Critical Care Ultrasound—Including FAST (Focused Assessment with Sonography in Trauma)

Role of ultrasound in the assessment and management of hemodynamic instability has been discussed.

RUSH PROTOCOL (RAPID ULTRASOUND IN SHOCK)

Evaluation of critically ill patients (hypovolemic/cardiogenic/obstructive shock)
It includes evaluation of
  Heart: Effusions and myocardial contractility
  Aorta: Dissections and aneurysms
  IVC: Volume status
Pleural fluid and pneumothorax
Fluid in the Morrison's pouch

FATE PROTOCOL (FOCUSED ASSESSMENT BY TRANSTHORACIC ECHOCARDIOGRAPHY)

Exclude any obvious pathology.
Assess wall thickness, contractility, and chamber dimensions (mainly eyeball technique is used).
Clinical correlation is imperative.

LEFT VENTRICULAR FAILURE

Mitral valve hitting the septum is a normal marker of the left ventricle function.
Dyskinetic septum suggests severely reduced left ventricular function.

RIGHT VENTRICULAR FAILURE

Normally RV < LV (two-third the size)

RV = LV (moderately enlarged size)
RV > LV (massive enlargement)

PERICARDIAL TAMPONADE

In a subxiphoid view, pericardial effusion in a patient with hypotension, tachycardia, and muffled heart sounds suggestive of right ventricular diastolic collapse.

PULMONARY EMBOLISM

Enlarged right ventricle.
McConnell's sign—right ventricular lateral wall akinesis along with apical sparing.

DEEP VEIN THROMBOSIS (DVT)

Paired superficial femoral and deep femoral arteries.
Deep femoral vein is not routinely seen on sonography due to small caliber.
Common femoral vein courses with paired femoral arteries.
Compressibility: Noncompressible femoral vein.
Augmentation: Normally vein fills with color and thrombus will not, on compressing distal part of the leg.

HYPERTROPHIC OBSTRUCTIVE CARDIOMYOPATHY WITH SYSTOLIC ANTERIOR MOTION OF MITRAL VALVE

Small left ventricular chamber
Proximal septal hypertrophy
Hypovolemia

BLUE PROTOCOL (BED-SIDE LUNG ULTRASOUND IN EMERGENCY)

Done for immediate diagnosis of acute respiratory
    failure. It is a fast protocol (<3 minutes); done
    in dyspnoeic patients admitted in ICU by an
    intensivist.
Lung ultrasound as described before (chest—
    Chapter 13).

FALLS PROTOCOL (FLUID ADMINISTRATION LIMITED BY LUNG SONOGRAPHY)

For management of acute circulatory failure.

FOCUSED ASSESSMENT WITH SONOGRAPHY FOR TRAUMA

A focused, goal-directed sonography examination
of the abdomen.

Goal is to detect the presence of hemoperitoneum/
    hemopericardium.
Part of initial survey of any patient with signs of
    shock or suspicion of abdominal injury.
Neither a definitive diagnostic investigation nor a
    substitute for CT.

Examines four areas for free fluid:

1. Perihepatic and hepatorenal space (Morisson's
    pouch)—RUQ view—probe is placed in right
    mid to posterior axillary line at level of 12th rib
    (Figure 14.1).
    Most dependent part of the upper peritoneal
        cavity.
2. Perisplenic space—LUQ view—Left posterior
    axillary line b/w 10th–11th ribs.
3. Pelvis—Most dependent portion of the lower
    abdomen where fluid will collect.

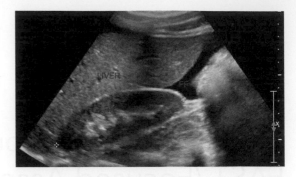

Figure 14.1 Illustrates free fluid in hepatorenal space.

    Probe is positioned midline just superior to
        symphysis.
4. Pericardial and pleural effusions—subxiphoid
    view for pericardial fluid between the fibrous
    pericardium and the heart seen as an anechoic
    collection around the heart.

Pleural effusion is seen as anechoic collection
    superior to echogenic diaphragm. In a stable
    patient, effusion can be visualized with the
    patient in sitting upright position.
Pericardial effusion is noted anterior to descend-
    ing aorta, pleural effusion will be posterior.

Quantification of hemoperitoneum: Scoring system.

Total score (0–8)
One point for each anatomic site in which free
    fluid is detected during the scan
Two points for fluid of ≥2 millimeters depth in
    hepatorenal/splenorenal space
One point for floating loops of bowel
Score >3 requires emergent management
Can detect 100–250 milliliters fluid
0.5 centimeter in Morrison's pouch—500 milliliters
1 centimeter—1,000 milliliters

Advantages

1. Rapid (2 minutes)
2. Portable
3. Inexpensive
4. Technically simple, easy to train
5. Serial scanning possible
6. Nonionizing, noninvasive
7. Useful for guiding triage decisions in trauma
    patients

Limitations

1. Does not typically identify the source of bleeding
2. Limitation in detecting bowel and mesentery pathology
3. Difficult to assess retroperitoneum
4. Requires extensive training to relatively assess parenchyma
5. Not able to detect <250 milliliters of intraperitoneal fluid
6. Limited in obese patients

EXTENDED FAST (e-FAST)

Includes bilateral hemithorax for

1. *Hemothorax*: Pleural fluid. Even ~20 milliliters can be detected.
2. *Pneumothorax*: Probe placed on the anterior chest third to fourth intercostal space in midclavicular line.

15

Acute Abdomen and Abdominal Tuberculosis

USG is advantageous because of its dynamic and real-time nature.

Can observe the presence or absence of peristaltic movements, blood flow pulsations, and fetal movements. Effects of valsalva, compression, and so on can be easily visualized.

High-frequency probe delineates the abdomen better. An expeditious evaluation—considering patient's age, gender, associated symptoms, duration, and location of pain—is imperative to rule out crucial pathologies requiring emergent management.

Most of the etiologies are discussed in the respective sections.

Etiologies:

1. Appendicitis.
2. *Perforated peptic ulcer*: Free fluid can be seen.
3. *Pelvic inflammatory disease (PID)*: Free air can be seen to collect between the liver and the lateral abdomen wall.
4. Adnexal lesion.
5. Ectopic pregnancy.
6. Ruptured aortic aneurysm.
7. Ureteral stone.
8. Renal colic.
9. *Crohns disease*: Marked thickening of bowel wall in a skip pattern.
   May be associated with focal discontinuity of the wall and a small walled-off abscess.
   Surrounding inflammation of fat, seen as hyperechoic noncompressible tissue adjacent to cecum. Mesenteric lymphadenopathy may be associated.
10. Infections ileocolitis/terminal ileitis.
    S/s—diarrhea, abdominal pain.

Diffuse thickening of terminal ileum and cecum.
Appendix appears normal.
Mesenteric lymphadenopathy.
11. Mesenteric lymphadenitis:
    Enlarged and inflamed mesenteric lymph nodes.
    Usually noted in childhood.
    Appendix appears normal.
12. *Caecal carcinoma*: Irregular asymmetric wall thickening.
    Associated with mesenteric lymphadenopathy.
    Look for metastasis in liver.
13. *Sigmoid/right-sided colonic diverticulitis*:
    Thickening of the wall of colon.
    Associated with guarding in left/right lower abdomen, fever, leucocytosis, and elevated ESR.
    Small paracolic abscesses may be seen.
    Considered as a medical emergency with recent onset of sudden and severe abdominal pain.
14. Urinary tract infection (UTI).
15. Liver abscess, hepatitis, cholecystitis, and biliary causes.
16. Pancreatitis.
17. Ruptured abdominal aortic aneurysm.
18. Miscellaneous causes such as lower lobe pneumonia, cardiac causes as myocardial infarction, gastritis, and intestinal obstruction.

ABDOMINAL TUBERCULOSIS

It affects mainly ileo-caecal junction (due to abundant lymphoid tissue), colon, liver, spleen, peritoneum, and lymph nodes.

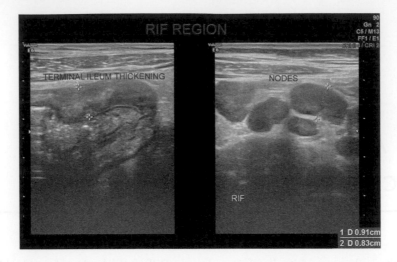

Figure 15.1 Illustrates terminal ileum thickening and lymphadenopathy.

USG FINDINGS

Ileocecal wall thickening (Figure 15.1)
Lymphadenopathy
Ascites—loculated/septated
Peritoneal thickening
Omental thickening
Intestinal obstruction
Matted loops of bowel

PERITONEAL TUBERCULOSIS

Wet ascitic type
Dry fibrous type
Liver, spleen: Multiple hypoechoic nodules.
S/S: Abdominal distension, weight loss, anorexia, fever, altered bowel habitus, anemia, and doughy abdomen.
Advise ascitic fluid examination, Mantoux test, culture sensitivity, and so on.
Most of the conditions have been discussed in their respective sections.

SUGGESTED READINGS

1. C. M. Rumack, S. Wilson, J. W. Charboneau, and D. Levine, *Diagnostic Ultrasound: 2-Volume Set*, Elsevier Health US, Philadelphia, 2010.
2. S. M. Penny, *Examination Review for Ultrasound: Abdomen & Obstetrics and Gynaecology*, Lippincott Williams & Wilkins, Philadelphia, PA, 2010.
3. W. Herring, *Learning Radiology: Recognizing the Basics*, Mosby Elsevier, Philadelphia, PA, 2007.
4. A. Adam, *Grainger & Allison's Diagnostic Radiology: 2–Volume Set*, Elsevier Health, London, UK, 2014.
5. C. M. Rumack and S. R. Wilson, *Diagnostic Ultrasound: Paediatrics*, Elsevier Health Sciences, Philadelphia, 2014.
6. D. Sutton, *Textbook of Radiology & Imaging, 2-Volume Set*, Elsevier, New Delhi, India, 2009.
7. S. G. Davies, *Chapman & Nakielny's Aids to Radiological Differential Diagnosis*, Elsevier Health-UK, 2014.
8. M. Hofer, *Ultrasound Teaching Manual: The Basics of Performing and Interpreting Ultrasound Scans*, Thieme, Stuttgart, Germany, 2005.
9. W. E. Brant and C. Helms, *Fundamentals of Diagnostic Radiology: 4-Volume Set*, Wolters Kluwer, Philadelphia, 2012.
10. W. Dahnert, *Radiology Review Manual*, Wolter Kluwer, Baltimore, 2011.
11. P. E. S. Palmer, B. Breyer, C. A. Brugueraa, H. A. Gharbi, B. B. Goldberg, F. E. H. Tan, M. W. Wachira, and F. S. Weill, *Manual of Diagnostic Ultrasound*, World Health Organisation, Geneva, Switzerland, 1995.
12. World Health Organization (WHO) and World Federation for Ultrasound in Medicine and Biology, *Manual of Diagnostic Ultrasound, Volume 1 & 2*, Geneva, Switzerland, 2013.

PART III

Obstetrics USG

16

Introduction

Routine history should be asked from the patient before starting the examination to make the patient comfortable.

1. Ask about last menstrual period (LMP).
2. Any symptoms concerning the patient such as pain, bleeding, and heaviness.
3. Previous obstetric history with details of abortions and types of previous delivery (vaginal/caesarean).
4. Previous USGs done so far.
5. Previous tests done (biochemical screening).

PREPARATION

<16 weeks: Full bladder is required.
TVS can be used preferably up to 12 weeks (with empty bladder).
16–24 weeks: Partially distended bladder is sufficient.
>24 weeks: No preparation is required.

If cervix and lower uterine segment have to be specifically evaluated, then full bladder assessment is required.

Empty stomach is not required for obstetric USG.

POSITION

TAS → patient lies supine on the bed with extended legs. Apply ample USG gel on the skin.
3.5–5 MHz transducer is sufficient for routine scanning by transabdominal sonography (TAS).
For TVS → 5–8 MHz transducer is used.

TVS: Patient should lie on her back in a gynecologic position with flexed hips and knees.

Clean TVS probe placed in an aseptic cover (Condom) with jelly inside the cover. Gel is then applied on the probe, which is then inserted into the vagina (anterior fornix) (Table 16.1).

Table 16.1 Illustrating fetal lie and presentation with respect to fetal spine

Lie	Presentation	Spine
Longitudinal	Cephalic	On maternal right. Fetus lying with its right side down
Longitudinal	Breech	On maternal left; fetus with its right side down
Transverse	Fetal head on maternal left	Fetal spine nearest the Lower uterine segment (LUS) with right side down
Transverse	Fetal head on maternal right	Fetal spine nearest the fundus with right side down

17

First Trimester

INTRODUCTION

Gestational period between conception and 13 weeks ±5 days

Nomenclature to be used:

Embryo <10 weeks
Fetus >10 weeks until delivery

Physiology

Pituitary gland secretes FSH and LH, which stimulates the growth of many primary follicles and a dominant (Graffian) follicle in the ovary due to estrogen stimulation.

Just before ovulation, progesterone and LH surge leads to formation of corpus luteum.

Corpus luteum secretes progesterone. If there is no pregnancy, corpus luteum involutes.

If pregnancy is positive, hCG maintains the corpus luteum and progesterone is responsible for decidual reaction.

Corpus luteum is the most common finding noted in the first trimester. Progesterone supports the pregnancy until the placenta can take over its hormonal process. May regress around 16–18 weeks of gestational age (GA).

Human chorionic gonadotropin (hCG) is a glycoprotein secreted by the outer layer of cells of gestation or chorionic sac (syncytiotrophoblasts). Negative hCG excludes the presence of live pregnancy. Beta-hCG levels in normal pregnancy can be detected about 11 days after conception by a blood test and 12–14 days after conception by a urine test. It has a doubling time of approximately 2–3 days. hCG levels begin to rise, reaching up to an average peak of 100,000 international units per liter; in the first 8–11 weeks of pregnancy.

Low levels suggest miscalculated dates, possible miscarriage, and ectopic pregnancy.

High levels suggest wrong dates, molar, and multiple pregnancies.

Indications

1. To identify the location and the number of the gestational sac (GS)
2. To assign a GA to the pregnancy
3. To evaluate normal early pregnancy
4. To look for any sonography indicators predicting failure
5. To assess maternal symptoms such as pain or bleeding
6. To evaluate uterine contents before the termination of pregnancy
7. To guide diagnostic/therapeutic procedures

USG APPEARANCES OF A NORMAL I/U GESTATION

Gestational sac

First USG sign to suggest early pregnancy.

Implantation commonly occurs in the fundal region of uterus between the 20th and 23rd day.

25–29 days of menstrual age (b-hCG +ve)→ Intradecidual sign (Small gestation sac within the decidua/focal echogenic thickening of endometrium at the site of implantation).

4.5–5 weeks menstrual age—Intradecidual sac (Normal GS).

Threshold level: Earliest we can expect to see a sac 4 weeks 3–4 days.

Discriminatory level: We should always see the sac at 5 weeks 3 days (Table 17.1).

Table 17.1 Illustrating presence of GS, YS, embryo, and cardiac activity at different gestational ages

GA	GS	YS	Embryo	Heart heat
5 weeks	+	–	–	–
5.5 weeks	+	+	–	–
6.0 weeks	+	+	+	+

DOUBLE DECIDUAL SAC SIGN (INTERDECIDUAL) (FIGURE 17.1A)

It is based on visualization of three layers of decidua in early pregnancy. There are two concentric echogenic rings surrounding a portion of GS.

Ring closest to the sac—Smooth chorion laeve and decidua capsularis.

Ring peripherally located—Decidua vera (echogenic endometrial lining).

Present when MSD >10 millimeters at 5–6 weeks GA.

Decidua basalis—Chorion frondosum forms future placenta—Seen as an area of eccentric echogenic thickening.

DOUBLE BLEB SIGN

On TAS at 5½ weeks, two blebs represent the amnion and yolk sac (YS).

Thin amniotic membrane divides amniotic and coelomic cavity.

Amniotic fluid fills in the amniotic cavity, which grows faster than the chorionic cavity and by 16 weeks, amniotic membrane is not seen as a separate structure.

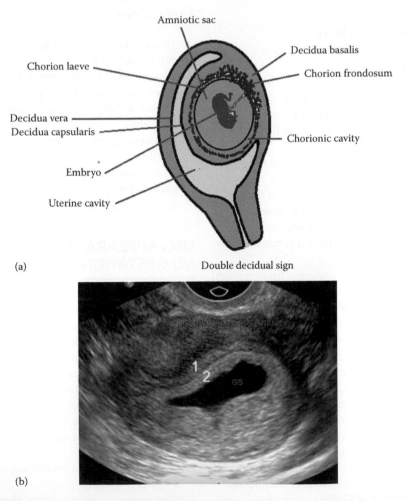

(a) Double decidual sign

(b)

Figure 17.1 (a) Illustrates double decidual sac sign (DDSS) and (b) illustrating two concentric rings of normal pregnancy.

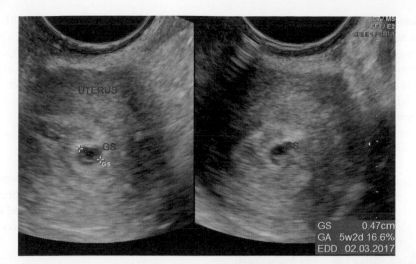

Figure 17.2 Illustrating small anechoic G sac in early pregnancy.

Gestational sac

Small round fluid collection surrounded by echogenic rim of tissue (Figure 17.2).

Normally, gestation sac is round in very early stages. As it enlarges, it has oval shape d/t pressure exerted by muscular uterine walls.

Mean sac diameter

Calculated by adding three orthogonal dimensions of the chorionic cavity (excluding the surrounding echogenic rim) and divided by three.

Yolk sac

First structure seen normally within the gestation sac, confirmatory of intrauterine pregnancy.

Round lucent structure with echogenic periphery, located in chorionic cavity outside the amniotic membrane (Figures 17.3 and 17.4).

Helps in

- Transfer of nutrients to the embryo
- Angiogenesis
- Hematopoesis

Using TAS: YS always seen with MSD of 20 millimeters

Using TVS: YS always seen with MSD of 8 millimeters

Number of YSs help in determining the amnionicity of the pregnancy.

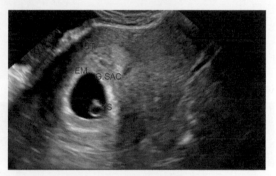

Figure 17.3 Illustrating yolk sac in early pregnancy.

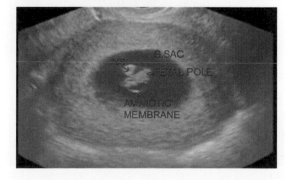

Figure 17.4 Illustrates early intrauterine pregnancy at around 7 weeks.

MCMA—Two embryos, one chorionic sac, one amniotic sac, and one YS.

DCDA—Two embryos, two chorionic sac, two amniotic sac, and two YS.

YS remains connected to the midgut by the vitelline duct (Omphalomesenteric duct [OMD]).

As the GA advances, YS separates and detaches from the embryo. Subsequently, its diameter decreases and is no longer detected by USG by the end of the first trimester.

Abnormal YS is also associated with early pregnancy failure.

Calcified, echogenic, double YS, and abnormally shaped YS are associated with pregnancy failure (Figure 17.5a and b). Follow-up is recommended.

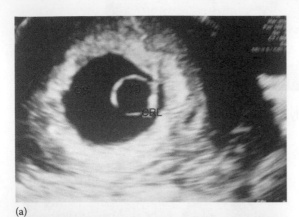

(a)

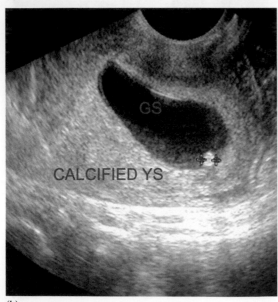

(b)

Figure 17.5 **(a)** and **(b)** Illustrating pregnancy failure with enlarged yolk sac or calcified yolk sac in two different patients.

Crown rump length (CRL) → CRL is the maximum straight line length of embryo/fetus in its longitudinal axis (Figure 17.6a). YS and extremities should not be included while calculating CRL, which increases by 1 millimeter per day between 6 and 10 weeks.

PLACENTA

- Starts developing around 8th week of GA.
- Echogenic ring around the sac becomes asymmetric with focal peripheral thickening of most deeply embedded portion of the sac.

6 weeks

- Shape of embryo changes from a flat disc into a C-shaped structure.
- Head size is almost half the total length of embryo.

7–8 weeks

- Limb buds appear.

10 weeks

- Visible hands and feet.
- Embryo becomes fetus (embryogenesis is completed); fetal cranium, neck, trunk, heart, bladder, stomach, and extremities can be visualized.

11 weeks

- Ossification is reliably seen. Swallowing starts at around 11 weeks.

12 weeks

- Placenta can be seen as granular gray appearance. Cord should insert into the central portion of the disc.

Amnion normally fuses with chorion at 12–16 weeks of gestation.

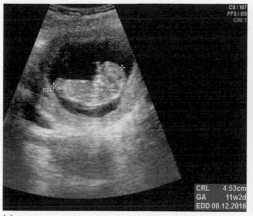 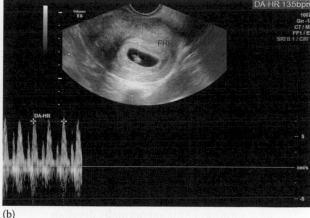

(a)   (b)

Figure 17.6 **(a)** Illustrating maximum straight length of fetus as CRL of 11 weeks 2 days and **(b)** Illustrates cardiac activity of embryo <6 weeks.

Fetal urine production begins at about 11–13 weeks. Renal dysfunction leading to oligohydramnios cannot be identified accurately before 16 weeks.

FETAL HEART RATE

<6 weeks—100–115 beats per minute
   (Figure 17.6b)
8 weeks—140–170 beats per minute
9 weeks—130–150 beats per minute

UMBILICAL CORD

Formed at the end of 6th week. It contains two umbilical arteries, one umbilical vein, the allantois, and yolk stalk (OMD/vitelline duct), which are embedded in the Wharton's jelly.

Embryonic demise (Early pregnancy failure)

Etiology:

1. Chromosomal abnormalities.
2. High maternal age, use of tobacco and alcohol → high frequency of morphologic abnormalities in preimplantation embryo.

3. *Luteal phase defect*: Failure of corpus luteum to adequately support the conceptus once implantation has occurred due to
   • Shortened luteal phase in cases of ovulation induction and IVF.
   • Luteal dysfunction in obese females and females aged >37 years.

USG features

1. *Cardiac activity*
   • Bradycardia <80 beats per minute in embryos with CRL <5 millimeters
     <100 beats per minute in embryos with CRL 5–9 millimeters
     <110 beats per minute in embryos with CRL 10–15 millimeters
   • Arrhythmias
   • Absence of cardiac activity
2. *Gestational sac*
   a. (MSD-CRL) <5 millimeters denotes small GS
   b. On *TAS*, GS is abnormal if
      MSD >10 millimeters without double decidual sac sign (DDSS)
      MSD ≥25 millimeters without an embryo

MSD ≥20 millimeters without YS
On TVS:
MSD >16 millimeters without embryo
MSD >8 millimeters without YS

c. Distorted GS shape
d. Thin trophoblastic reaction (<2 millimeters)
e. Weakly echogenic trophoblast
f. Abnormally low position of GS within the endometrial cavity

3. *Amnion and YS criteria*:
   a. >7 weeks maternal age (MA)—Visualization of amnion in the absence of embryo evinces its resorption (Amnion normally develops after the embryo).
   b. Collapsing irregularly marginated amnion.
   c. YS calcification (a/w abnormal outcome) versus solid echo dense YS (live embryo). YS malformations occur in embryos of diabetic mothers in the first trimester of pregnancy <9 weeks. At 8–12 weeks, YS <2 millimeters is associated with poor outcome.
   d. On TVS—MSD >8 millimeters nonvisualization of YS.
   e. Nonvisualization of YS in the presence of embryo.
   f. At 5–10 weeks—YS diameter >5.6 millimeters.
   g. Abnormal large YS—Associated with chromosomal abnormalities (trisomy 21), partial molar pregnancy, and omphalocele.

4. *Low serum beta HCG*
5. *Subchorionic hemorrhage* (intrauterine blood collections near the GS) leading to elevation of chorionic membrane d/t:
   • Abruption of placental margin
   • Or marginal sinus rupture
     Acute—Hyper to isoechoic to placenta.
     1–2 weeks—Sonolucent.
6. *Amniotic sac abnormalities*:
   Larger than normal/floppy amniotic sac.

Guidelines

1. Blighted ovum
   On TVS, GS of MSD >20 millimeters with no evidence of an embryo or YS (Figure 17.7).
2. Missed abortion
   Embryo of CRL >7–10 millimeters without cardiac activity on two separate occasions of at least 7 days apart.
   If MSD <15 millimeters or CRL <10 millimeters, then the examination should be repeated 2 weeks later to assess growth of GS and embryo and any evidence of cardiac activity.
3. If GS < expected for GA, possibility of incorrect dates should always be considered, especially when there is no pain or bleeding. Repeat TVS after a period of 7 days.

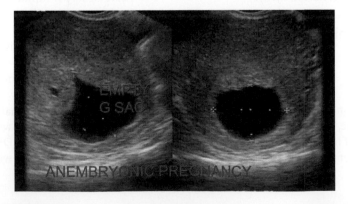

Figure 17.7 Illustrating blighted ovum with empty gestational sac with no yolk sac or embryo.

ABORTION

Spontaneous abortion—Termination of pregnancy <20 weeks of GA

Recurrent abortion—≥3 consecutive spontaneous abortion

Absent I/U sac

D/D

1. Early spontaneous abortion
2. Very early I/U pregnancy
3. Ectopic pregnancy

Correlate with hCG levels and follow-up ultrasound scans.

I/U sac without an embryo/yolk sac

D/D

1. Normal early intrauterine pregnancy (IUP)
2. Abnormal IUP
3. Ectopic pregnancy with pseudogestational sac

Follow-up USG is required to verify the subsequent appearance of YS/embryo.

Table 17.2 Illustrating chronology of yolk sac and cardiac activity on TVS and TAS

		YS (evident)	Cardiac activity
TVS	GA	5.4 weeks	6–6.3 weeks
	MSD	8 millimeters	13–19 millimeters
TAS	GA	7 weeks	8 weeks
	MSD	20 millimeters	26 millimeters

Thickened/irregularly echogenic endometrium

1. I/U bleed
2. Retained products of conception after an incomplete spontaneous abortion
3. I/U GS—Located within decidua
4. Pseudogestational sac—Located in the uterine cavity

TVS should be done preferentially to evaluate I/U fluid collection, cardiac activity, early YS, and embryo detection, if any doubt per abdomen (Table 17.2).

Table 17.3 Illustrating varying USG presentation in different types of abortion

Term	Presentation	USG
Threatened abortion	Vaginal bleeding Internal os closed	• Embryo with cardiac activity • Empty GS that subsequently develops with embryo • Empty uterus
Complete abortion	Complete passage of gestational tissue	Empty uterus
Incomplete abortion	Incomplete passage of gestational tissue	• Thickened and irregular endometrium (retained products—endometrial blood and trophoblastic tissues with abnormal GS) • Fluid in the endometrial cavity
Abortion in progress	Bleeding with clots and cramps	GS in the process of expulsion
Embryonic (fetal demise)	Lack of FHR Lack of uterine growth	Discrete embryo without cardiac activity
Blighted ovum (anembryonic pregnancy)	Lack of FHR	Discrepancy in GS development and embryonic development with little or no embryonic remnant

FIRST TRIMESTER COMPLICATION

1. Vaginal spotting/frank bleeding—temporary and self-limited.
2. Abortion.
3. Entities presenting as threatened abortion are ectopic pregnancy and gestational trophoblastic disease (GTD). Monitoring with serum hCG level is required (Table 17.3).

TERMINATION OF PREGNANCY

Medical termination: Mifepristone (600 milligrams) followed by misoprostol (400 micrograms) 2 days later.
Surgical: Suction dilatation and curettage (D&C) under local anesthesia.

FIRST TRIMESTER SCREENING FOR ANEUPLOIDY

1. *Nuchal translucency*
   Measurement of collection of fluid under the skin behind the fetal neck.
   In midsagittal section, fetus should be in a neutral position and horizontal on the screen.
   Only the fetal head and upper thorax should be included in the image.
   Maximum magnification should be done.
   More than one measurement should be taken.
   Normally, the thickness should be <3 millimeters at ~11–12 weeks (Figure 17.8)
2. *Nasal Bone* at 11–14 weeks
   Midsagittal view with probe held in parallel to the direction of nose (Figure 17.9)
   Normally, three distinct lines seen
   Top—*Skin*
   Thick, echogenic line—*Nasal bone*
   Bottom line—In continuity with the skin but higher (*the tip of nose*)

The first two horizontal and parallel lines proximal to forehead resemble an *equal sign*.

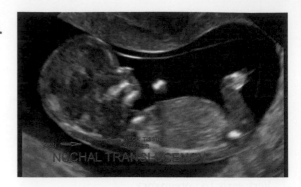

Figure 17.8 Illustrating normal nuchal translucency at 12 weeks.

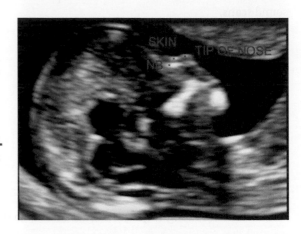

Figure 17.9 Illustrating equal sign of skin and nasal bone.

Normal embryologic development simulating pathology

1. The earliest cystic structure normally visualized in the posterior fossa region might be mistaken for posterior fossa cyst is actually normal embryonic *rhombencephalon*, which later forms normal 4th ventricle.
2. At 8th week of gestation, midgut normally herniates into umbilical cord—rotates 90 degrees counterclockwise—Returns to the abdomen during the 12th week.

This *physiological herniation of anterior abdominal wall* appears as small echogenic mass protruding into the cord. Follow-up should be done after 12 weeks.

18

Second Trimester

NORMAL USG

Indications of USG

1. *Gestational age estimation*: Based on biparietal diameter (BPD), head circumference (HC), femur length (FL), and abdominal circumference (AC) by comparing these parameters to the reference curves. If difference between maternal age (MA) and gestational age (GA) >2 weeks, pregnancy should be redated.

   BPD: Measured in the transverse plane from the outer edge of the near temporoparietal bone to the inner edge of the far temporoparietal bone. Thalamus should be visualized at this level (Figure 18.1).

   HC: Outer-to-outer diameter is measured at the same level (Figure 18.1).

   AC: Measured in the transverse plane at the fetal liver with the umbilical portion of left portal vein in the center of the abdomen (Figures 18.1 and 18.2).

   Normal heart rate should always be measured (Figure 18.2).

2. *Fetal morphology assessment*: Requires systematic scanning.

3. *Amniotic fluid volume*

   By measuring the deepest pocket fluid in each of the four quadrants and adding the four values.

   If >20 centimeters—Polyhydramnios

   <5 centimeters—Oligohydramnios

4. *Placenta*:

   Location of placenta

   Umbilical cord evaluation

   Distance of placenta to internal os

5. *Presentation and cardiac activity of fetus*

6. *For invasive procedures*

   Level-1 examination: Standard or routine obstetric ultrasound—Includes evaluation of the maternal uterus, cervix, adnexa, placenta, and fetal anatomy.

   Level-2 examination: Specialized/targeted obstetric ultrasound—Detailed fetal anatomic survey that should be done by an expert in obstetric imaging.

Fetal morphology assessment

1. *Head*:

   Measurement of BPD and HC with assessment of CSP, thalami, third ventricle, and sylvian fissure (*Transthalamic plane*).

   Atrial width (~7.5 millimeters is normal and >10 millimeters is abnormal)—Thickness of the atrium of lateral ventricles (*Transventricular plane*).

   Transverse diameter of the cerebellum with assessment of vermis, cisterna magna (4–10 millimeters depth), and fourth ventricular (*Transcerebellar plane*).

   Orbital morphology and symmetry (*Transorbital plane*).

   Fetal brain scanning is done in four planes.

2. *Vertebral column* (Spine)
   - Longitudinal scanning along the entire vertebral column.

3. *Chest*: Display of
   - Lungs
   - Cardiac situs
   - Four-chamber view
   - Left ventricular outflow tract (LVOT)
   - Right ventricular outflow tract (RVOT)

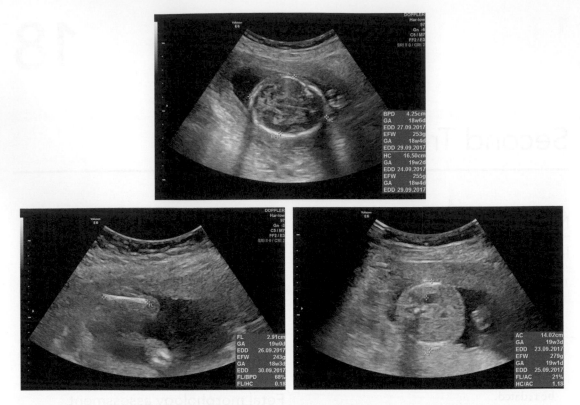

Figure 18.1 Illustrating BPD, head circumference (HC), and abdominal circumference (AC) at 16 weeks 4 days.

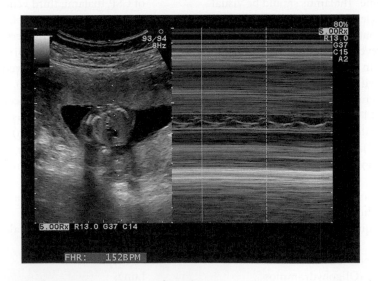

Figure 18.2 Illustrating fetal cardiac activity of 152 beats per minute at 16 weeks 4 days.

4. *Abdomen*
   Measurement of AC (the plane with stomach and portal vein).
   Visualization of stomach, anterior abdominal wall, bladder, and kidneys.
   Normal fetal kidneys can be visualized on TAS around 12 weeks.
5. *Extremities*: Mainly the presence and length (morphology) of long bones of the four limbs. FL is accurate when it shows two blunted ends.

CHROMOSOMAL ABNORMALITY (GENETIC) SCREENING

Trisomy 21 (Down syndrome)

SONOGRAPHIC MARKERS

Major markers

Thickened nuchal fold
Hypoplastic/absent nasal bone
Flattened facies
Cardiac defects
Duodenal atresia
Ventriculomegaly, brachycephaly
Reversed flow in ductus venosus

Minor markers

Short femur and humerus, clinodactyly of the fifth finger
Echogenic intracardiac focus
Echogenic bowel
Pyelectasis
Sandal toes—Exaggerated gap between the first and second digits

BIOCHEMICAL MARKERS

First trimester

High free beta-hCG (b-hCG)
Low pregnancy-associated plasma protein A (PAPP-A)

Second trimester

Quadruple screening

1. Alpha-fetoprotein (AFP)
2. Unconjugated estriol (uE3)
3. Inhibin
4. b-hCG

Trisomy 18 (Edward's syndrome)

IUGR with polyhydramnios
CNS abnormalities—Strawberry-shaped skull, choroid plexus cyst, abnormal cerebellum, and cisterna magna
Neural tube defects
Cardiac defects
Omphalocele
Clenched hands with overlapping index fingers, syndactyly, and club foot

Trisomy 13 (Patau's syndrome)

CNS defects—Holoprosencephaly. Dandy walker, ventriculomegaly, and microcephaly
Facial clefts
Neural tube and cardiac defects
Postaxial polydactyly
Echogenic kidneys
Ocular malformations

Turners syndrome (45 XO)

Septated cystic hygromas
Hydrops
Cardiac defects

19

Third Trimester

FETAL BIOMETRY

Fetal measurements and estimated fetal weight (EFW) can be compared with previous measurements of the same fetus to longitudinally evaluate the growth.

BPD and head circumference (HC) are measured in the axial plane of fetal head (Figure 19.1).

Abdominal circumference (AC) is measured where the transverse diameter of the liver is greatest (Figure 19.2).

This is considered the most variable and most difficult measurement.

FL—Whole femur diaphysis excluding proximal and distal epiphysis in a plane approximately 90 degrees to the USG beam.

AMNIOTIC FLUID EVALUATION

Subjective assessment: Involves the comparison of anechoic fluid areas surrounding the fetus with the area occupied by the fetus and placenta.

Objective assessment: Maximum vertical pocket (MVP)—Measuring the single deepest amniotic fluid pocket free of umbilical cord and fetal parts.

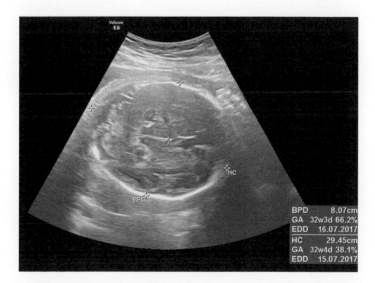

Figure 19.1 Illustrating BPD and HC in the third trimester.

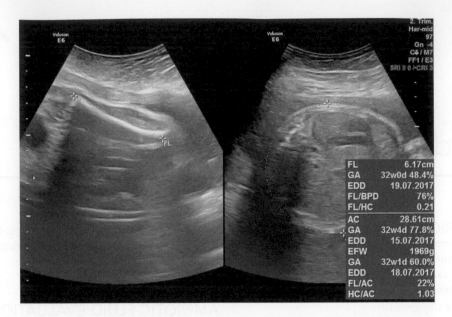

Figure 19.2 Illustrating abdominal circumference and femur length in the third trimester.

Amniotic fluid index (AFI): Sum of the deepest AF pockets measured in the four quadrants of the gravid uterus.

Amniotic fluid (AF) volume begins to decline near term in postterm women.

EFW: Optimal ranges are 3,000–4,000 grams.

Macrosomia: >4,000 grams. Associated with high risk of maternal and fetal trauma, shoulder dystocia with Erb's palsy. Perinatal asphyxia, meconium aspiration, and post-partum haemorrhage (PPH).

Usually noted in infants of diabetic mothers.

20

Fetal Malformations

HEAD

1. *Anencephaly*: Absence of fetal calvaria, no parenchymal tissue seen above the orbit (bulging orbits, mimicking frog's eyes), and incompatible with life. Elevated maternal serum alpha-fetoprotein (MSAFP) (Figure 20.1).
2. *Microcephaly*: Fetal head and brain are smaller than normal.
3. *Macrocephaly*: Enlarged fetal head d/t severe hydrocephalus or presence of intracranial masses (tumors/cysts).
4. *Cephalocele*: Protrusion of meninges alone—*Meningocele.*
   Of meninges and brain tissue—*Encephalo meningocele* through a bony defect located in the occipital pole usually (Figure 20.2).
5. Ventriculomegaly (Hydrocephalus) (Figure 20.3).

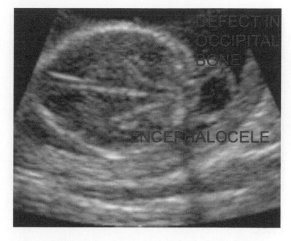

Figure 20.2 Depicting occipital encephalocele.

   Atrial width <10 millimeters—normal
   10–15 millimeters—Borderline
   >15 millimeters—Severe ventriculomegaly.
6. *Choroid plexus cysts*: Usually B/L (Figure 20.4)
   Transient and disappears by the end of second trimester (TM). Cystic collection in B/L ventricles.
7. Holoprosencephaly
   Alobar: Horseshoe shape of single ventricle with fused thalami.
   Semilobar: Frontal horns are fused with abnormal occipital horns.
   Lobar: Difficult to diagnose.
8. Dandy–Walker complex (DWC) (Figure 20.5)
   DWC (Complex) classic
      Severe hypoplasia of vermis
      Enlarged fourth ventricle a/w hydrocephalus
   Dandy walker variant (*DWV*) (*variant*)
      Mild hypoplasia of vermis

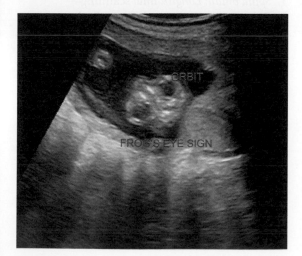

Figure 20.1 Illustrates frog's eye sign of anencephaly.

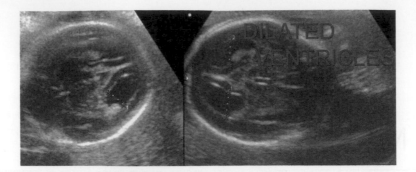

Figure 20.3 Illustrating hydrocephalus.

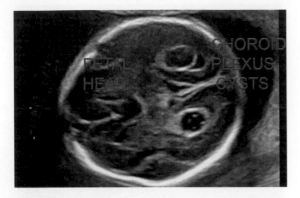

Figure 20.4 Illustrating bilateral choroid plexus cysts.

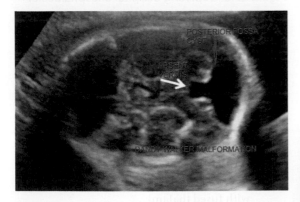

Figure 20.5 Illustrating Dandy–Walker malformation with posterior fossa cyst and absence of vermis.

Enlarged fourth ventricle with key-hole appearance
D/D Blake pouch cyst—Normal vermis.
9. *Mega cisterna magna*: Anteroposterior (AP) diameter at the level of cerebellar vermis >10 millimeters.

10. *Chiari II*: Small posterior fossa, effaced cisterna magna, and banana-shaped cerebellum. Lemon-shaped calvaria.
11. At the level of orbits →
    a. Hypotelorism
    b. Cyclopia
    c. Hypertelorism
    d. Microphthalmia
    e. Anophthalmia

FETAL SPINE

Three ossification centers, one for vertebral body anteriorly and two for laminae are visualized in the transverse section of the spine. They appear like three dots of two eyes and one nose (Figure 20.6).

Longitudinal view to demonstrate the integrity of spinal canal (Figure 20.7).

1. *Spina bifida*: *Longitudinal* scanning— Enlargement at the level of vertebral defect. *Axial*—Lateral displacement of laminae.

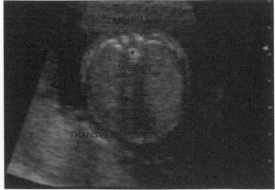

Figure 20.6 Depicts normal spine in the transverse section.

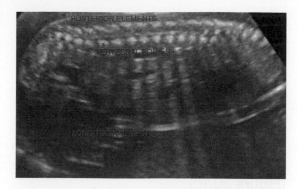

Figure 20.7 Illustrating normal fetal spine in longitudinal view.

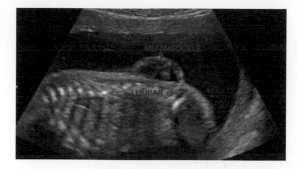

Figure 20.8 Illustrating lumbar meningocele.

Meningocele—Cystic structure protruding from vertebral defect (Figure 20.8).
2. *Sirenomelia (Caudal regression syndrome)*: Variable degree of agenesis of spine and pelvis. Single/fused lower extremity. A/w single umbilical artery (SUA), renal agenesis (marked oligohydramnios), and imperforate anus.

FETAL LUNGS

Axial view—Seen as echogenic wings surrounding the fetal heart.

1. *CCAM*: U/L (Congenital cystic adenomatoid malformation)
   Part of the lung tissue is replaced by dysplastic cystic tissue.
   Microcystic: Too small cysts.
   Macrocystic: Cysts can be visualized as an echogenic area in the lung.
   Small: Spontaneous regression may occur
   Large: Mediastinal shift seen
2. *Sequestration*: Aberrant pulmonary tissue that does not communicate with the normal bronchial tree/pulmonary vessels.

On CDUS—Feeding vessel can be visualized directly originating from the descending aorta.
3. *Pleural effusion*: Anechoic fluid collection in the pleural cavity compressing the fetal lung.
   U/L—Can be chylothorax.
   B/L—Can be d/t heart anomalies, infections, lung anomalies, and hydrops.
4. *Diaphragmatic hernia*: Abdominal organs protrude into the mediastinum through diaphragmatic defect with contralateral mediastinal shift.

FETAL HEART

Four-chamber view of the heart can be (Figure 20.9)

Apical: When the apex of fetal heart points anteriorly toward the transducer.
Transverse: When the cardiac axis is perpendicular to the USG beam.

Proper acquisition of four-chamber view requires

1. Normal situs in relation to stomach.
2. Two-third of the heart is in left half of the thorax.
3. Apex toward left (Levocardia).

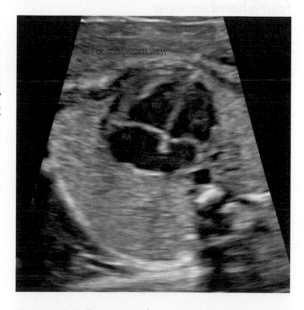

Figure 20.9 Illustrating four-chamber view of fetal heart.

4. At least two pulmonary veins noted opening into the left atria.
5. Similar sized atria.
6. Foramen ovale discontinuity in the atrial septum.
7. Tricuspid valve inserted slightly lower than the mitral valve.
8. Almost same size of wall thickness of ventricles but different shape.
   Left ventricle (LV): Elongated and reaches the apex
   Right ventricle (RV): Circular (due to moderator band)
9. No breach in interventricular septal (IVS).
   Left ventricular outflow tract (*LVOT*)
       From the four-chamber view.
       Rotate the transducer slightly toward the right fetal shoulder.
       Ascending aorta originating from the LV.
   Right ventricular outflow tract (*RVOT*)
       Similar movement toward left fetal shoulder.
       Pulmonary artery originating from RV and crossing the aorta.
Three-vessel plane: Axial section of superior venacava (SVC), aorta, and pulmonary artery; posterior to thymus from four-chamber view, moving the transducer upward.

Anomalies detected with four-chamber view

1. *Atrial anomalies*:
   a. Single atrium (in AV canal)
   b. Enlarged RA (Ebstein's anomaly)
   c. Enlarged LA (due to Mitral Stenosis)
2. *Septal defects*: Larger defects can be visualized.
3. Ventricular disproportion:
   a. Small LV (Hypoplastic left heart) due to mitral atresia
   b. Small RV (Tricuspid atresia)
   c. RV hypertrophy (due to coarctation of aorta)
   d. LV dilatation (critical aortic stenosis)

Anomalies diagnosed in outflow tract

LVOT: IVS defects
RVOT: Aorta overrides the defect
    Small pulmonary artery
    Pulmonary artery arising directly from the aorta

Fetal gastrointestinal tract (Figure 20.10)

Normal in axial view:

Upper section
• Echo-free stomach
• Echogenic liver with intrahepatic umbilical vein
• GB
Lower section
• Echogenic bowel
1. *Esophageal atresia*—Lack of visualization of stomach.
   a/w polyhydramnios.
   If Tracheoesophageal fistua (TEF)—Partial filling of the stomach.
2. *Duodenal atresia*: Dilation of stomach and proximal duodenum.
   a/w polyhydramnios.

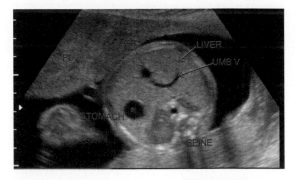

Figure 20.10 Illustrating normal fundic bubble, liver, and intrahepatic portion of umbilical vein.

3. *Ileo-jejunal obstruction*: Multiple cystic areas in the abdomen below the liver due to dilatation of intestinal lumen.
4. *Omphalocele*: Abdominal defect at the level of insertion of the umbilical cord.
   Protruding loops/organs are covered by membrane.
   Cyst of Wharton's jelly seen at the insertion site.
   Associated with anomalies, hence worse prognosis.
5. *Gastroschisis*: Defect is on the right side of the cord insertion.
   Not covered by membrane.
   Loops float freely in the amniotic cavity.
6. *Ascites*: Increased AC due to fluid-filled abdomen cavity.

GENITOURINARY TRACT ANOMALIES

Axial view helps in demonstrating normal kidneys (Figure 20.11) and bladder.

Normal renal pelvis is dilated maximum up to 5 millimeters.

1. *B/L renal agenesis*:
   Nonvisualization of kidneys and bladder.
   Associated with oligohydramnios.
   Absence of renal arteries.

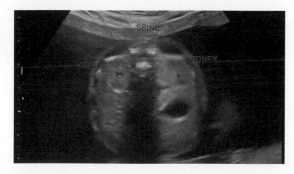

Figure 20.11 Illustrating normal fetal kidneys bilaterally.

2. *PCKD*: Polycystic kidney disease.
   B/L enlarged and hyperechoic kidneys.
   Severe oligohydramnios.
3. *MCDK*: Multicystic dysplastic kidney.
   U/L with enlarged affected kidney d/t the presence of multiple cysts of varying sizes.
4. *Posterior urethral valve (PUV)*
   Due to prolonged lower urinary tract obstruction.
   Common in males.
   Markedly distended bladder and ureter with B/L hydronephrosis (key-hole appearance).
   Oligohydramnios and pulmonary hypoplasia.
5. *Urinary tract obstruction*
   High level: Pelvi-ureteric junction (PUJ) stenosis—Graded dilatation of renal pelvis and calyces with the thinning of renal parenchyma.
   Middle level: uretero-vesical junction (UVJ) stenosis/primary megaureter— Hydroureteronephrosis of varying degree.
   Lower urinary tract—PUV with vesicoureteric reflux (VUR), urethral atresia—Dilated bladder with bilateral hydronephrosis.
   Key-hole appearance may be noted.

SKELETAL SYSTEM

Long bones and extremities

Rhizomelia—Affecting femur, humerus
Mesomelia—Tibia, fibula, radius, and ulna
Acromelia—Hand, foot
Micromelia—Total hypoplasia
Abnormally curved hypoplastic bones
Shortening and bowing of bones (Telephone receiver configuration)
Club foot

Spine and chest

Abnormal spine due to scoliosis or hemivertebra.
Hypoplastic chest (a/w lung hypoplasia)— Neonatal death.

Head

Synostosis → Abnormal shape. Most common
   is cloverleaf skull in thanatophoric dysplasia
   (Figure 20.12)
Frontal bossing
Micrognathia

Degree of mineralization

Hypomineralization → thin and transparent bones
a/w osteogenesis imperfecta and hypophosphatasia.

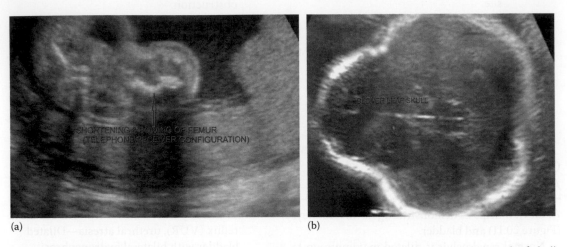

(a)   (b)

Figure 20.12 **(a)** and **(b)** Illustrates telephone receiver configuration of long bones and cloverleaf skull in thanatophoric dysplasia.

21

Placenta

INTRODUCTION

At USG, the placenta may be visible as early as 10 weeks as a thickening of the hyperechoic rim of tissue around the gestational sac.

Fetal placenta—Chorion frondosum—develops from the blastocyst
Maternal placenta—Decidua basalis—develops from maternal uterine tissue
At 12–13 weeks, blood flow is easily demonstrable
By 14–15 weeks—Placenta is well established
  Prominent hypoechoic retroplacental area composed of decidua, myometrium, and uterine vessels
Normal-term placenta measures 15–20 centimeters in length and 400–500 grams in weight at term
  Maximum—4–5 centimeters in thickness
Thin placenta—Small for date fetus
  Sign of intrauterine growth retardation (IUGR)
Thick placenta (Placentomegaly)
  Homogenous thickening

1. Diabetes mellitus (Gestational)
2. Anemia
3. Hydrops
4. Infections
5. Aneuploidy

Heterogenous (With multiple cystic spaces)

1. Triploidy
2. Placental hemorrhage
3. Villitis
4. Mesenchymal dysplasia
5. Beckwith–Wiedmann syndrome

Placental Grading—Grannum classification (Figures 21.1 and 21.2)

Grade 0—Homogenous placenta, uniform echogenicity—first and early second trimester
Grade 1—Occasional hypo-/hyperechoic areas—late second trimester
Grade 2—Larger calcifications along the basal plate—early third trimester
Grade 3—Larger and denser calcifications along with compartmentalization of placenta—late third trimester

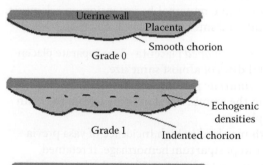
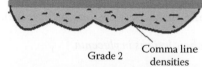
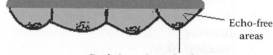

Figure 21.1 Illustrates grading of placental maturity.

117

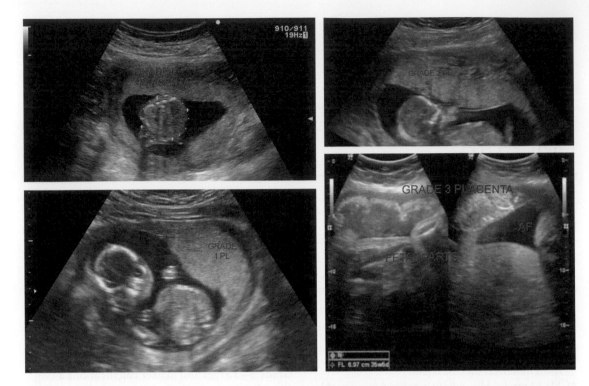

Figure 21.2 Illustrates varying grades of placental maturity in a normal fetus.

Premature/accelerated calcifications have been a/w chronic maternal hypertension preeclampsia, IUGR, and smoking.

Bipartite/Bilobed placenta—Two separate placental discs of almost same size.

Succenturiate placenta—Accessory lobe develops in the membrane at a distance from the main placenta.

Both may lead to high incidence of vasa previa and postpartum hemorrhage, if retained.

Circumvallate placenta—Chorionic plate (on fetal side) is smaller than basal plate (on maternal side).

Cystic/Hypoechoic lesions in placenta

1. Intervillous thrombus—1–2 centimeters in diameter
2. Decidual septal cysts—<3 centimeters in diameter
3. Placental lakes

Clinically less significant, unless a/w Rh incompatibility and elevated maternal serum alpha-fetoprotein (MSAFP).

Placental hematomas—Hypoechoic area with the absence of flow (Figure 21.3).

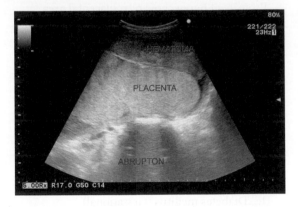

Figure 21.3 Illustrating retroplacental hematoma.

1. Subchorionic/marginal
2. Preplacental/subamniotic
3. Retroplacental

When small in size, clinically they are less significant.

Abruption

Large retroplacental hematomas with elevation and detachment of posterior placenta from the uterine wall s/o abruption.

Patient presents with sudden abdominal pain with vaginal bleeding.

D/D—Hypoechoic fibroid and uterine contractions.

Abnormal adherence of placenta to the uterus may not separate after delivery of the fetus.

Predisposed due to previous C-section and placenta previa.

Types

Placenta *accreta*—Villi penetrate the decidua, but not the myometrium

Placenta *increta*—Villi penetrate the decidua and myometrium, but not the serosa

Placenta *percreta*—Villi penetrates the myometrium, serosa, and may be adjacent organs such as the bladder

Hemorrhage

Acute	(0–48 hours)	Hyperechoic
Subacute	3–7 days	Isoechoic
Chronic	1–2 weeks	Hypoechoic
	>2 weeks	Anechoic

Placenta previa

Placenta proximate to the internal cervical os (Figure 21.4).

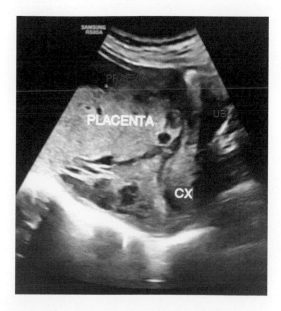

Figure 21.4 Illustrating placenta previa covering the os.

Most common cause of bleeding in the third trimester.

Low-Lying Placenta—Extends into lower uterine segment (LUS), usually >2 centimeters from the internal os and does not cover or reach it. Should be evaluated with partially full bladder. Overdistension may lead to apposition of anterior and posterior LUS, leading to false appearance of placenta previa. Reevaluation is required after emptying the bladder.

Marginal Placenta—Reaches the edge, but does not cover the internal os.

Partial Previa—Placenta partially covers the dilated internal os.

Central Previa—Mid portion of placenta, not just the edge, completely covers the os.

Complete Previa—Portion of the placenta completely covers the os.

Overly distended maternal bladder or a transient myometrial contraction of LUS can potentially mimic a true placenta previa. Patient should always be evaluated postvoiding if there is suspicion of placenta previa.

Chorioangiomas

MC benign neoplasm of the placenta.

On USG:

- Well-circumscribed, round, and hypoechoic/heterogenous mass near the umbilical cord insertion site on the fetal surface of the placenta (Figure 21.5).
- Moderate vascularity.
- D/D hematoma, subchorionic fibrin deposition, and adjacent degenerating leiomyoma.

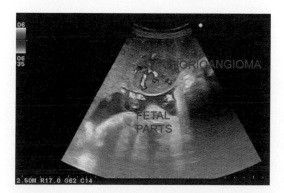

Figure 21.5 Demonstrates chorioangioma of placenta.

22

Amniotic Fluid

INTRODUCTION

Volume of amniotic fluid (AF) represents a balance between

1. Mechanisms producing AF—fetal urine flow, oronasal, and lung secretions
2. Mechanism allowing passage of fluid into the amniotic cavity—fluid movement through the chorion frondosum and membranes, highly permeable fetal skin
3. Mechanism involved in uptake of AF—fetal swallowing

   Fetal urination is the major source of AF in the second half of pregnancy

   Increase in intramembranous absorption of AF leads to decrease in AFV in cases with chronic severe placental insufficiency

   Echogenic AF is the presence of particles in amniotic fluid (represent either meconium or vernix)

   Usually not associated with any adverse pregnancy outcome

Functions

1. It cushions the fetus against physical trauma.
2. Allows for capacious growth of the fetus without any distortion by adjacent structures.
3. Imparts thermally stable environment.
4. Helps to prevent infection.
5. Source of nutrients to the developing embryo.

Amniotic fluid index technique

Divides the uterus into four quadrants using maternal sagittal midline vertically and transverse line approximately halfway between symphysis pubis and uterine fundus (Figure 22.1).

Select the deepest AF pocket free of umbilical cord and fetal parts. The greatest vertical dimension is measured with USG transducer perpendicular to the floor.

(Maximum vertical pocket [MVP])
>2 centimeters—normal
—1–2 centimeters—reduced
<1 centimeter—oligohydramnios
>8 centimeters—polyhydramnios

Process is repeated in each of four quadrants eight pocket measurements added = AFI.

If AFI <8 centimeters, perform the four-quadrant evaluation 3 times and average the values.

Stumbling blocks in correct estimation of amniotic fluid volume

1. Shift in fetal position alters the measurement of amniotic fluid volume (AFV).
   AFI may appear higher for fetuses lying centrally within the uterus in comparison with fetuses lying laterally within the uterus.
2. Pseudoreduction in AFI as a consequence of excessive maternal abdominal transducer pressure.
3. Umbilical cord filled with AF pocket should not be used in the assessment of AFV. Doppler imaging assists in identifying the cord.

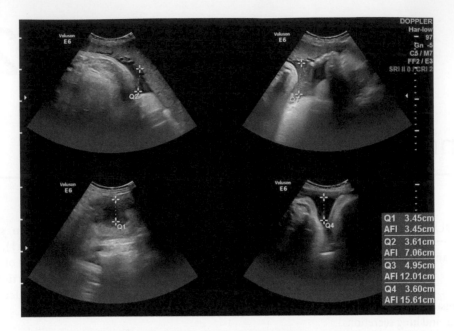

Figure 22.1 Illustrating technique measuring amniotic fluid index.

4. Fat scatters the ultrasound beam and may introduce artifactual echoes into AF. Obese patients may have low fluid because of artifactual echoes.

   Use of low-frequency transducer helps in the correct estimation of AFV.

5. In the third trimester, free floating particles due to vernix makes the true amniotic space less conspicuous.

OLIGOHYDRAMNIOS

Condition in which AFV is reduced.
AFV <300–500 milliliters after the midtrimester.
Maximum vertical pocket <1–2 centimeters.
AFI <5 centimeters.

Causes

1. Urinary tract abnormalities—such as B/L renal agenesis, posterior urethral valves, Potter's sequence, and so on.
2. IUGR due to uteroplacental insufficiency.
3. PROM—Preterm rupture of membranes.
4. Postterm pregnancy.
5. Drug induced (prostaglandin inhibitors, angiotensin converting enzyme [ACE] inhibitors).

Amnion nodosum—associated with severe oligohydramnios, pulmonary hypoplasia, and renal agenesis.

USG

Lack of fluid (Figure 22.2)
Crowding of fetal parts
Poor fluid fetal interface
Increased risk of pulmonary hypoplasia

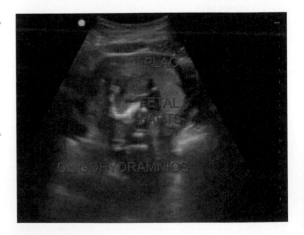

Figure 22.2 Scanty amniotic fluid with crowded fetal parts.

POLHYDRAMNIOS

Excessive accumulation of amniotic fluid with floating fetal parts (Figure 22.3).

AFV > 1,500–2,000 milliliters.

Deepest vertical pocket > 8 centimeters.

AFI > 24 centimeters.

Acute → appear within days; usually occur in the second trimester.

Chronic → occurs gradually in the third trimester.

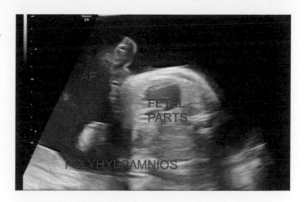

Figure 22.3 Illustrating excessive amniotic fluid.

Causes

1. Maternal diabetes mellitus.
2. Erythroblastosis fetalis.
3. GIT abnormalities such as esophageal and duodenal atresias.
4. CNS abnormalities—anencephaly and so on.
5. Cardiovascular abnormalities.
6. Musculoskeletal abnormalities.

Congenital mesoblastic nephroma and U/L ureteropelvic junction obstruction may be a/w polyhydramnios.

23

Umbilical Cord and Biophysical Profile

INTRODUCTION

Anatomy

First visualized at 8 weeks as a straight thick structure, when diameter <2 centimeters.

Umbilical artery arises from fetal internal iliac artery. In newborn, it becomes the superior vesical artery and the medial umbilical ligament.

Umbilical vein carries oxygenated blood from the placenta to the fetus through ductus venosus into IVC and to the heart.

Single left umbilical vein becomes ligamentum teres and attaches to the left portal vein.

Ductus venosus becomes the ligamentum venosum in newborns.

Allantois is associated with bladder development, becomes urachus and median umbilical ligament.

Yolk stalk connects the primitive gut to yolk sac. The paired vitelline vessels follow the stalk to provide blood supply to the yolk sac.

Cord normally inserts in the central portion of the placenta. May insert marginally and paramarginally.

Velamentous insertion—Insertion of cord beyond the edge into the free membrane.

Vasa previa—Fetal vessels running across the internal os of the cervix. Inadvertent rupture of vessels during spontaneous labor may prove fatal. Plan C-section.

Average length of the cord—59 centimeters (22–130 centimeters)

Short cord may be a/w aneuploidy, extreme IUGR, and so on.

Excessive cord length a/w asphyxia due to excessive coiling, true knots, cord prolapse, and multiple loops of nuchal cord.

Normally contains two arteries and one vein. Vessels of the cord are surrounded by Wharton's jelly.

Single umbilical artery (SUA), cord cysts, hernias, hematomas, and masses should be excluded.

Nuchal cord

Entanglement of the umbilical cord around the fetal neck (Figure 23.1).

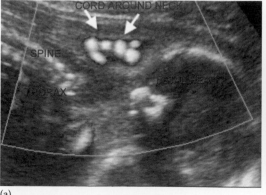
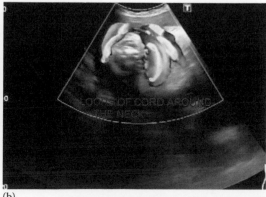

(a)   (b)

Figure 23.1 **(a)** and **(b)** illustrating cord loops around the neck.

Single loop of umbilical cord seen near the fetal neck is an incidental finding and less a/w fetal jeopardy.

Two loops of cord posterior to neck/circumferentially, best seen with color Doppler. If a/w oligohydramnios, IUGR, postdate pregnancy, and decreased fetal movements, require close surveillance and caesarean delivery sometimes.

BIOPHYSICAL PROFILE—BPP (MANNING SCORE)

Normal two score for each with a total of 10. Score between 8–10 is considered normal (Table 23.1).

Table 23.1 Illustrating biophysical profile

Fetal breathing	At least 1 episode for 30 seconds in 30 minutes
Fetal movements	At least 3 movements of limbs/spine in 30 minutes
Fetal tone	At least 1 extension of limb/spine coming back to flexion in 30 minutes
Fetal heart rate (NST—nonstress test)	Two episodes of acceleration of 15 beats per minute for >15 seconds
Amniotic fluid index (AFI)	Normal AFI score is >6

24

Gestational Trophoblastic Neoplasia

INTRODUCTION

Includes

- Hydatidiform mole—Complete hydatidiform mole (CHM) and partial hydatidiform mole (PHM) (Table 24.1)
- Invasive mole (chorioadenoma destruens)
- Coexistent complete mole and live fetus
- Choriocarcinoma
- PSTT—Placental site trophoblastic tumor

Presentation

Vaginal bleeding
Uterine enlargement more than expected for gestational age (GA)
Abnormally high hCG levels
Prevaginal passage of vesicles
Low levels of maternal serum alpha-fetoprotein (MSAFP)

IMAGING

USG

Enlarged uterine cavity filled with heterogeneous mass with cystic spaces of varying sizes (BUNCH OF GRAPES appearance) (Figure 24.1)

- No fetal development in complete mole.
- B/L theca—lutein cysts in enlarged ovaries.
- Myometrial invasion is seen in cases of invasive mole.
- Heterogeneous mass with areas of necrosis and hemorrhage is s/o choriocarcinoma.

Diagnosis

Gold study is histopathological examination.
Immunohistochemistry.

Beta-hCG levels are higher than expected. High levels persist for >6 months after molar evacuation.

Table 24.1 Illustrating differentiation between complete and partial mole

Complete mole	Partial mole
Almost always diploid (46XX)	Almost always triploid (69XXY)
Due to both overexpression of paternally transcribed and loss of maternally transcribed genes	Due to overexpression of paternally transcribed genes
No fetal tissue and diffuse placental changes	Fetal tissue with patchy cystic changes in placenta
Sperm fertilization of an empty ovum	Normal ovum fertilized by two sperms

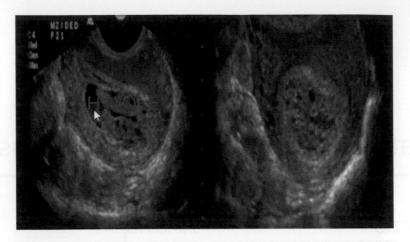

Figure 24.1 Illustrating hydatidiform mole in an enlarged uterus.

Reliable contraception should be recommended while hCG levels are being monitored.

Choriocarcinoma

Aggressive, rapid growth.
Vaginal bleeding, high HCG levels.
USG—enlarged uterus; echogenic solid mass with small cystic spaces in the endometrial cavity. Theca lutein cysts.
Hemorrhage, necrosis, vascular invasion, and distant metastasis common. CXR should always be advised.

Placental site trophoblastic tumor

Slow growing, fatal

Resistant to chemotherapy
Human placental lactogen (HPL) positive

Invasive mole

Chorioadenoma destruens

Management

Uterine suction evacuation rather than sharp curettage to decrease the risk of perforation.
Follow-up with serial hCG measurements for identification of persistent gestational tropho-blastic neoplasia (pGTN) (Persistent) cases. Chemotherapy may be required in some cases.

Ectopic Pregnancy

25

Definition: Pregnancy that occurs outside the uterine cavity.

Classical clinical triad: Seen only in 45% of cases
Pain
Abnormal vaginal bleeding
Palpable adnexal mass
Other S/s:
Amenorrhea
Adnexal tenderness
Cervical excitation tenderness

RISK FACTORS

1. Any tubal abnormality
2. Previous tubal pregnancy
3. H/o tubal reconstructive surgery
4. Pelvic inflammatory disease (e.g., *Chlamydia salpingitis*)
5. Intra-uterine contraceptive device (IUCD)
6. Maternal factors (increasing age and parity)
7. Previous C-section

Heterotopic

- Coexistent intrauterine and ectopic
- Increase risk in multiple pregnancies with ovulation induction and IVF
- Correlation with β-hCG levels should be done

USG

1. Empty uterus with decidual cast or pseudoges-tational sac is seen
   Intrauterine fluid collection/IU sac filled with low-level echoes surrounded by a single decidual layer (Figure 25.1)
   (c.f. two concentric rings of double decidual sign in intrauterine pregnancy)

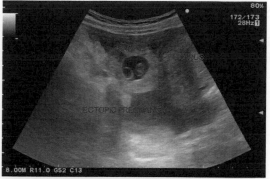
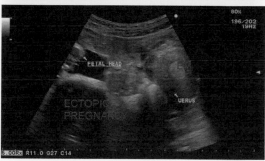

Figure 25.1 Illustrating ectopic pregnancy outside the uterine cavity.

2. Adnexal tenderness
3. Large/complex mass (may be extrauterine G sac/hematoma)
4. Free fluid in hepatorenal space (S/o urgency to the surgeon)
5. Live embryo in the adnexa
6. Ectopic tubal ring
   - Concentric ring created by trophoblast of ectopic pregnancy surrounding the chorionic sac.
   - Ring is often seen within a hematoma that may be confined to the fallopian tube or may extend outside.

- It is more echogenic.
- Peritrophoblastic flow—High velocity, low resistance flow with low resistive index (RI) and pulsatility index (PI).

D/D:

a. Corpus luteum cyst—Located eccentrically within the rim of ovarian tissue Less echogenic
b. Bowel
c. Hydrosalpinx

7. *Hemoperitoneum*: Echogenic-free fluid in pelvis or blood clots in posterior cul-de-sac

Site

Implantation in the cornua of the endometrial canal is normal. It extends into the endometrial canal within a week.

1. Ampullary/isthmic portion of the fallopian tube.
2. Interstitial (intramural)—embryo is implanted *lateral* to the round ligament.
   Ruptures later.

Causes massive intraperitoneal hemorrhage with a high mortality.
Interstitial line sign—Thin echogenic line extending from endometrial canal up to the cornual sac/hemorrhagic mass.

3. Cervical scar implantation.
   Painless vaginal bleeding with a h/o previous C-section.
   Sac implanted in lower uterine segment (LUS) with local thinning of myometrium.
4. Angular pregnancy—Rare type of cornual (nearly ectopic) pregnancy. Embryo is implanted in the lateral angle of uterine cavity, *medial* to uterotubal junction and round ligament. Can progress to term or miscarriage may occur.
   Other—ovarian, abdominal—rare sites.
5. Management.
   Laparoscopy is used for definitive diagnosis.
   Conservative surgical procedures—salpingotomy.
   Surgical—resection of diseased tube.
   Medical management—Methotrexate (iv/im/oral—decreased β-hCG levels).

26

Multifetal Pregnancy

Dizygotic twins

Arise from two separate fertilized ova (Zygotes) (Figure 26.1).
Each embryo with its own amnion, chorion, and yolk sac.
Dichorionic/diamniotic (DC/DA) twin pregnancy.
Two placentas or one fused placenta.

Monozygotic: Arise from the division of a single zygote.

DC/DA

Division of zygote during first 3 days of postconception.
Two embryos with two amnions and two chorions.
Two placenta or one fused placenta.

MC/DA

Division occurs b/w 4–8 days postconception.
Two embryos, two amnions, and two yolk sacs within a single (one) chorion.
Single placenta.

MC/MA

Division after day 8 of postconception.
Two embryos within a single (one) amnion and single (one) chorion.

Conjoined twins

Incomplete division of embryonic disc.
Division of embryonic disc after day 13 of postconception is usually incomplete.

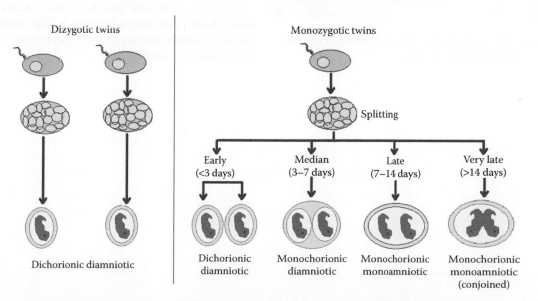

Figure 26.1 Illustrating splitting of zygote into different types of twin pregnancies.

In dichorionic twins, there is thick septum between the chorionic sacs.

Lambda/chorionic peak sign: Thick septum between the two chorionic sac and extension of thick placenta into this intertwin membrane (Figure 26.2).

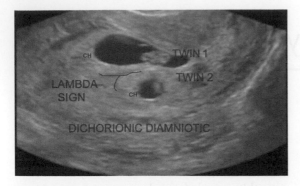

Figure 26.2 Illustrating lambda/chorionic peak sign in dichorionic pregnancy.

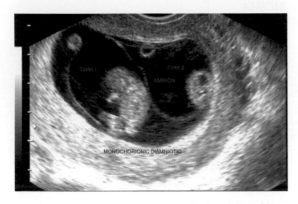

Figure 26.3 Illustrating T sign in monochorionic diamniotic twin pregnancy.

T Sign

S/o MC/DA twins

Two opposed thin amniotic membranes forming T-shaped junction when they abut the middle of placenta (Figure 26.3).

MC/MA: Absence of intertwin membrane.

TWIN–TWIN TRANSFUSION SYNDROME

Serious complication of monochorionic gestation (fused placenta) with growth discordance.

Interconnecting placental vessels between two twins leading to umbilical arteriovenous shunting of blood from one twin to another.

One twin (donor)—small, anemic, oligohydramnios

Other twin (recipient)—large, polyhydramnios, volume overload, heart failure

TWIN REVERSED ARTERIAL PERFUSION SEQUENCE (ACARDIAC—PARABIOTIC TWIN)

Seen in monochorionic gestation.

Intraplacental arterial–arterial and venous–venous connections.

One fetus is normal and the other is acardiac (amorphous tissue mass) creating a large cardiovascular burden leading to polyhydramnios and heart failure in normal fetus.

Hydrops and Intrauterine Fetal Death

Abnormal accumulation of serous fluid in at least two body cavities or tissues.

USG

Fetal ascites, pleural, and pericardial effusions.
Subcutaneous edema, scalp, and body-wall edema (Figure 27.1).
Placentomegaly.

Causes

Immune—Rh alloimmunization.
Nonimmune—Others such as CVS, GIT, and maternal causes.

Rh isoimmunization—Fetal RBCs leak into maternal circulation. Maternal anti-Rh IgG antibodies form, crosses the placenta and leads to hemolysis of fetal Rh RBCs (Erythroblastosis fetalis).

INTRAUTERINE FETAL DEATH ON USG

Death of fetus after 20 weeks of pregnancy. Before 20 weeks, it is termed as miscarriage.

Signs

1. Absence of fetal heart rate (FHR)
2. Absence of fetal movements
3. Spalding's sign—Overlapping of skull bones (Figure 27.2)
4. Soft tissue edema (skin thickness >5 centimeters)—Also known as Deuel's sign (Halo sign)
5. Macerated fetus
6. Robert sign—Gas shadow in fetal heart

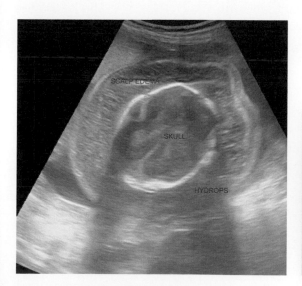

Figure 27.1 Illustrating scalp edema in a patient with hydrops.

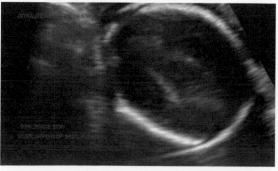

Figure 27.2 Illustrating overlapping of skull bones in a patient with intrauterine fetal death.

28

Incompetent Cervix

INTRODUCTION

Cervix appears as a soft tissue structure with medium-level echoes

Endocervical canal appears as echogenic line (mucus plug) surrounded by hypoechoic zone of endocervical glands

Cervical length: Normal cervix is >3 centimeters in length (length of endocervical canal from the internal os to the external os)

Cervical width: Anteroposterior (AP) diameter of the cervix at the midpoint between internal and external os

Gradual cervical effacement and shortening normally begins at ~30 weeks of gestation.

In multifetal pregnancy, cervix is much shorter from 20-week gestation onward.

Widening of os and cervical length <2.5 centimeters at </= 24 weeks is s/o cervical insufficiency.

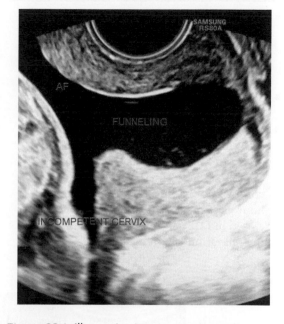

Figure 28.1 Illustrating incompetent cervix.

IMAGING

USG findings

- *Funneling* of the internal os has been reported as an early sign (Figure 28.1).
  Seen as a bulging/herniation of fetal membranes >3 millimeters into the internal os.
  >50% funneling before 25 weeks is a/w >75% risk of preterm delivery.
- *Shortening* of cervical canal (from internal os to external os).
- Cervical canal gets dilated and in severe cases, amniotic sac may prolapse through (Figure 28.2) the cervix into vagina with or without the products of conception. (*Bulging amnion*).

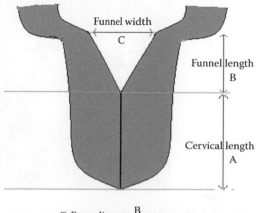

$$\% \text{ Funneling} = \frac{B}{A + B}$$

Figure 28.2 Illustrating cervical measurements.

135

Narrowing of prolapsed sac by an incompletely dilated cervix leads to *hour glass*.

Shape of amniotic sac on ultrasound (US).

Increased risk of preterm delivery

Cervical stress test—Leads to early diagnosis of cervical incompetence. Application of mild fundal pressure induces funneling and dilatation that were otherwise not present.

STUMBLING BLOCKS

- Distended bladder compresses the cervix and obliterates the fluid within the endocervical canal, masking the true cervical dilatation and leading to false cervical elongation.
- Hypoechoic cervical canal may be mistaken with the herniated membranes.
- Cervix incompetence is a dynamic process. Therefore, cervix should be continuously observed for several minutes.
- Sometimes lower uterine segment (LUS) contraction may give a false appearance of hour glass membrane. However, internal os is closed in LUS contraction. Repeat scan after the relaxation of contraction.

MANAGEMENT

Cervical cerclage by applying a purse string suture to the cervix using Shirodkar and Mac Donald technique.

On transvaginal sonography (TVS), cervical length <2.5 centimeters is a cut off for intervention.

MISCELLANEOUS

Uterine fibroids

Fibroids may be seen in pregnant females. May lead to first-trimester bleeding as a complication. If multiple, they may block the birth passage and increase the risk of premature labor and necessitate caesarean section. May also lead to miscarriage.

Focal myometrial contraction (Braxton–Hicks contractions)

Seen as transient thickness of a focal region of myometrium, simulating a fibroid. May last for seconds or minutes or hours before resolving. Review scan should be done to look for resolution of focal myometrial contraction (Figure 28.3).

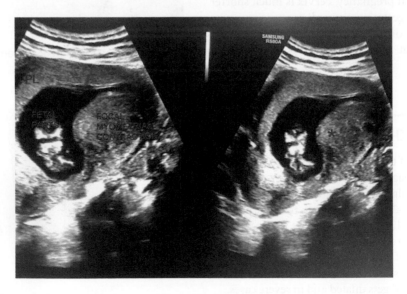

Figure 28.3 Illustrating myometrial contraction, simulating fibroid.

Scar thickness

Planning vaginal birth after caesarean (VBAC) is the difficult choice and depends on the scar thickness of the previous caesarean section (C-section).

It is measured in the midsagittal plane along the LUS most efficiently when the head of the fetus gets engaged (>36 weeks).

Thinnest zone of LUS is measured at the urinary bladder–myometrial interface. Thickness of LUS decreases with advancing gestation. The *cut off* of scar thickness after a previous C-section is 3.5 millimeters.

Risk of rupture is proportional to thinning of the segment.

Luteal phase defect

Leads to early pregnancy failure.

Occurs due to failure of corpus luteum to adequately support the conceptus once the implantation has happened.

Defined as a delay of >2 days in histological development of endometrium relative to the day of cycle.

Etiology: Shortened luteal phase due to ovulation induction and IVF. Obese and age >37 years are the risk factors.

Findings

Low FSH/LH

Low/Abnormal pattern of hormone production by corpus luteum.

Reduced response of endometrium to progesterone.

Intraovarian artery in nongravid females during luteal phase.

In normal females—RI <0.47.

In females with luteal phase defect—RI >0.5.

29

Infertility

Defined as couple's inability to conceive after 1 year of unprotected intercourse

Primary—When the patient has never conceived.
Secondary—When there is h/o previous
  conception.

OVARY

Factors need to be considered are

1. Ovarian follicular development
2. Ovulation
3. Formation of functional corpus luteum
4. Associated ovarian pathologies such as benign cysts (simple/complete dermoid/fibromas)

Follicular monitoring: Best done by transvaginal sonography (TVS):

Spontaneous cycles
Induced cycles

From 10th day of menstrual cycle, observe the developing/dominant follicle with the concurrent assessment of circulating estrogen levels. Predict impending ovulation. (Presence of cumulus oophorus)

Ovulation occurs on ≅ 14th day of menstrual cycle in a 28-day cycle. Suggested by follicle rupture with crenated follicular walls with evacuation of follicular fluid and cumulus/oocyte complex with fluid in Pouch of Douglas (POD).

Corpus luteum develops after ovulation in normal cycle.

Corpus luteum cyst—2.5–4 centimeters diameter.

Corpus hemorrhagicum—Blood-filled corpus luteum.

Corpus albicans → hyperechoic structure in the ovary.

Growth of corpus luteum is proportional to luteal vascularity and serum progesterone concentration.

Causes

1. Absence of dominant follicle/or preovulatory follicle with low estrogen concentration
2. Ovulation failure

Failure of rupture of preovulatory follicle with extrusion of oocyte/cumulus complex with thick walls. (LUF syndrome—Luteinized unruptured follicle syndrome)

Capillaries in the follicular wall fenestrate and extravasate blood into the follicular lumen. (HAF—Hemorrhagic anovulatory follicle)

Correlate with basal body temperature (BBT) and midcycle progesterone levels.

Ovarian endometriomas—Functional endometrial
  tissue in ovary.
On USG—circumscribed cystic lesion with homogeneous low-level echoes.
Dermoid cysts—Heterogeneous mass with
  Rokitansky nodule (tip of iceberg).

PCO morphology

- Ovarian volume >9–11 cubic centimeters in asymptomatic patients.
- >10–12 follicles, 2–8 millimeters in size, peripherally placed (String of pearls/necklace sign) Graffian follicles in arrested stage of low FSH.
- High stromal echogenicity and may be a/w endometrial thickening in the uterus.

Table 29.1 Illustrating severity of OHSS with ovarian size

Severity	Mild	Moderate	Severe
Ovarian size	>5 centimeters	5–10 centimeters	>10 centimeters with large cysts

Multifollicular ovaries:

Chaotically distributed multiple follicles.
Irregular ovulatory pattern as in premature menopause, postmenarchal/premenopausal state.
Seen in patients recovering from anorexia.
Mildly enlarged ovaries.

Ovarian hyperstimulation syndrome (OHSS):
Complication of ovulatory induction with gonadotropins. Associated with pleural and pericardial effusion (Table 29.1).

NORMAL SPONTANEOUS CYCLE

On USG: Developing follicles of size ~3–5 millimeters can be illustrated.

7 days before LH surge → 1–2 follicles develop to ~10 millimeters and 1 dominant follicle takes over.
5 days before ovulation → dominant follicle grows at the rate of—2–3 millimeters per day.
Just before ovulation → reaches up to 17–25 millimeters diameter.

INDUCED CYCLES

Cycles are induced in

1. Patients with infertility d/t anovulation.
2. Patient with normal ovulation before assisted conception techniques in vitro fertilization–embryo transfer/gamete intra fallopian transfer (IVF–ET/GIFT) to increase the number of oocytes aspirated.

Cycles are induced by clomiphene citrate and human menopausal gonadotropin (hMG).
From 10th day of menstrual cycle—Patient is examined every alternate day.
Patients undergoing IVF–ET → from 7th–8th day of cycle—USG is done daily to monitor follicular development.
TVS is best to predict optimal time for administering ovulation-inducing dose of hCG.

hCG is best administered once follicles reach 15–18 millimeters.

UTERUS

Anatomic—Adhesions, congenital malformation, and leiomyomas.
Physiological—Lack of normal endometrial response to hormonal stimulation.

1. *Endometrial adhesions/synechiae*: Echogenic bridges in endometrial cavity or irregularities of endometrium surrounded by cystic spaces.
2. *Fibroids* (Leiomyoma): Heterogeneous hypoechoic lesions with calcifications/cystic areas with recurrent shadowing.
   If located in cornua → Occludes intramural portion of oviduct.
   If the contour of uterine cavity is altered → They may affect implantation.
3. *Endometrium Polyps*: Hypoechoic mass in the endometrium cavity a/w feeder vessel.
4. *Adenomyosis*: Marked heterogeneous myometrium with cystic changes and venetian blind shadowing. No abnormal vascularity seen.
5. *Nontuberculous chronic endometritis*: Thin echogenic endometrium that does not thicken as follicular phase advances.
6. *Endometrium ossification*: Highly reflective echogenicity on USG; acts like IUCD.

TUBAL FACTOR (OVIDUCT/FALLOPIAN TUBE PATHOLOGY)

Usually not visualized normally because of the surrounding bowel. Hysterosalpingography (HSG) is better to visualize oviduct in females with patient fallopian tube (FT).

Fallopian tubes transfer sperm from uterus toward ampulla
Conducts ova from the fimbriated end to the ampulla

Supports early embryo
Transfers embryo from the ampulla into the
uterus for implantation
Normal 8–15 centimeters length

Most common cause of infertility → Tubal pathology

1. Tubal obstruction d/t infection, endometriosis
2. Salpingitis isthmica nodosa (SIN)—Multiple
   small diverticulae in proximal 2/3 of tube
3. Tubal spasm (Cornual portion of tube is
   encased by smooth muscle of uterus.)
   Spasmolytic agent → Muscle relaxation →
   　　Tube opacification on HSG
4. TB Salpingitis—a/w calcified lymph nodes
5. Hydrosalpinx—Distended tube → Cystic,
   hypoechoic retort-shaped appearance with
   incomplete septations
   Pyosalpinx—Peritubal adhesions → adnexal
   　　loculated fluid collections.

Congenital malformation—Mullerian developmental anomalies mullerian duct anomalies (MDA)
a/w renal and vertebral anomalies. Kidneys and
skeleton should also be evaluated.

1. *Agenesis/hypoplasia*—Mayer Rokitansky
   Kuster Hauser (MRKH) syndrome
   Hypoplastic uterus shows normal relation
   　　between the length of cervix and that of
   　　the uterine body, whereas infantile uterus
   　　shows larger cervix than the uterine body.

2. *Unicornuate uterus*
   a/w spontaneous abortion and premature labor
   a/w poorest fetal survival
   　　Without rudimentary horn
   　　With rudimentary horn on contralateral side
   　　– Communicating
   　　– Noncommunicating → endometrial
   　　　　tissue is expelled retrogradely with
   　　　　high frequency of endometriosis.
   Difficult to diagnose on USG. Can be confused
   　　as a small mass.
3. *Uterine didelphys*—a/w highest possibility of
   successful pregnancy.
4. *Uterine bicornuate* (Figure 29.1)
   ● Intercornual distance >4 centimeters.
   ● Concavity of fundal contour with >1
   　　centimeter indentation
   ● Obtuse angle >105 degrees
   ● a/w incompetent cervix
   　　Serial scanning is required during pregnancy
   Unicollis—Septum extends up to internal os.
   Bicollis—Septum extends up to external os.
5. *Septate*—Most common
   ● Intercornual distance <4 centimeters
   ● Contour normally convex with <1 centi-
   　　meter indentation
   ● Acute angle <75 degrees
   ● Treatment is septoplasty via hysteroscopy.
   ● Associated with reproduction failure.
   MRI is better to differentiate these anomalies.
6. *Arcuate uterus* → No effect on fertility.
7. *Diethylstilbestrol (DES) exposure in utero.*

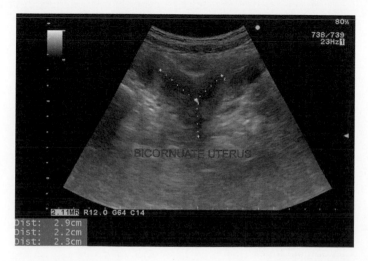

Figure 29.1 Illustrating bicornuate uterus.

Pre-Conception Pre-Natal Diagnostic Techniques Act

India first enacted PNDT act in 1994, later amended as pre-conception pre-natal diagnostic techniques (PCPNDT) act in 2003.

An act with a provision for the prohibition of sex selection (before or after conception), and for regulation of prenatal diagnostic techniques preventing their misuse for sex determination leading to female feticide in India.

Rules:

1. No person shall convey the sex of the fetus to the pregnant lady or her relatives by words, signs, or any other method.
2. Mandatory registration of all the machines and diagnostic laboratories by the appropriate authority.
3. Form F should be aptly filled and submitted to appropriate authorities by the 5th day of each following month.
4. All records should be maintained for minimum of 2 years period and made available for inspection by appropriate authorities.
5. USG machine should not be sold to anyone who is not registered under the act.
6. Certificate of registration shall be nontransferable. In the event of change of ownership, new owner shall apply afresh for the grant of certificate of registration.
7. Certificate of registration shall be valid for a period of 5 years.
8. Sign board "Disclosure of sex is prohibited under law" shall be displayed in both English and local language in the room and hospital premises.

Form A—Application for registration/renewal of registration of a genetic counseling centre, genetic laboratory, and genetic clinic.

Form B—Certificate of registration.

Form C—Rejection of application for registration or renewal of registration.

Form D—Record to be maintained by the genetic counseling centre.

Form E—Record to be maintained by the genetic laboratory.

Form F—Record to be maintained by the genetic clinic/USG clinic/imaging centre (name, address, registration number, and full record of the pregnant lady).

Form G—Form of consent for invasive techniques.

Form H—Maintenance of permanent record of application for grant or rejection of registration or renewal under the PNDT act.

SUGGESTED READINGS

1. P. W. Callen, *Ultrasonography in Obstetrics and Gynecolgy*, 6th ed, Elsevier, Philadelphia, PA, 2016.
2. C. M. Rumack, S. Wilson, J. W. Charboneau, and D. Levine, *Diagnostic Ultrasound: 2-Volume Set*, 4th ed., Elsevier Health-US, 2010.
3. S. M. Penny, *Examination Review for Ultrasound: Abdomen & Obstetrics and Gynaecology*, Lippincott Williams & Wilkins, Philadelphia, PA, 2010.

4. W. Herring, *Learning Radiology: Recognizing the Basics*, Mosby Elsevier, Philadelphia, PA, 2007.

5. A. Adam, *Grainger & Allison's Diagnostic Radiology: 2-Volume Set*, Elsevier Health-UK, 2014.

6. D. Sutton, *Textbook of Radiology & Imaging: 2-Volume Set*, Elsevier, New Delhi, India, 2009.

7. S. G. Davies, *Chapman & Nakielny's Aids to Radiological Differential Diagnosis*, Elsevier Health-UK, 2014.

8. M. Hofer, *Ultrasound Teaching Manual: The Basics of Performing and Interpreting Ultrasound Scans*, Thieme, Stuttgart, Germany, 2005.

9. W. E. Brant, and C. Helms, *Fundamentals of Diagnostic Radiology: 4-Volume Set*, Wolters Kluwer, Alphen aan den Rijn, the Netherlands, 2012.

10. W. Dahnert, *Radiology Review Manual*, Wolter Kluwer, Alphen aan den Rijn, the Netherlands, 2011.

11. P. E. S. Palmer, B. Breyer, C. A. Brugueraa, H. A. Gharbi, B. B. Goldberg, F. E. H. Tan, M. W. Wachira, and F. S. Weill, *Manual of Diagnostic Ultrasound*, World Health Organisation, Geneva, Switzerland, 1995.

12. World Health Organization (WHO) and World Federation for Ultrasound in Medicine and Biology, *Manual of Diagnostic Ultrasound*, Volume 1 and 2, 2013.

PART IV

Color Doppler

31

Basic Terminology

INTRODUCTION

Discovered by Christian Johann Doppler in 1842. Color Doppler (CD) is used for detection of blood flow in the vessels.

Doppler shift—Change in frequency of sound waves when there is relative motion between the source and the reflector.

No relative motion of target toward or away from the transducer is detected at an angle of 90 degrees; therefore, no Doppler shift is detected.

$$\text{Velocity} = \text{frequency} \times \text{wavelength}$$

If an object moves away from the transducer, wavelength increases and frequency decreases (Figure 31.1).

Rayleigh scattering—Occurs when a target is smaller in size than wavelength of incident sound beam. No reflection returns to the transducer. For example, scattering from moving RBCs in color Doppler studies.

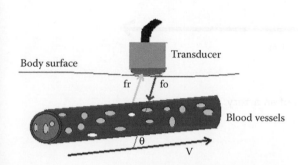

Figure 31.1 Illustrating color Doppler principle.

Types

Continuous Wave (CW) Doppler—Sound wave is continuously transmitted from one piezoelectric crystal and received by separate transducer. Can detect and record even very high-frequency shifts. Depth resolution is not possible.

Pulse Wave (PW) Doppler—Sound wave is alternately transmitted and received using only one crystal. Depth of echo source can be detected. Intensity of PW Doppler is more than CW Doppler.

Spectral Doppler—Represented by a graph of flow with time.

Duplex imaging—B mode + PW Doppler.

Flow directed **a**way from transducer is usually encoded **B**lue. Flow directed **t**oward the transducer is usually encoded **R**ed (TRAB). Colors can also be changed.

- Faster velocities are displayed in brighter colors.
- Generally, color in the upper half of the scale is s/o flow *toward* the transducer and color in the lower half of the scale is s/o flow *away* from the transducer.

  Sample volume (SV) is a box positioned in the centre of the vessel lumen. Depicts the area of movement being scanned. Width of the SV should not be >two-thirds of the vessel diameter.

  Doppler angle should be between 45 degrees and 60 degrees.

  Spectral broadening represents chaotic movement of blood cells leading to flow disturbances and multiple velocities filling up the spectral window. Very high Doppler gain settings and sampling close to the wall may lead to artifactual spectral broadening.

Wall filter—Device to suppress very slow flow near the baseline. It eliminates the artifacts caused by low-frequency pulsation of the vessel wall.

Pulse repetition frequency (PRF)—Number of transmitted pulses per second.

High-flow velocity vessels require high PRF setting.

Slow flow (venous) velocity vessels require low PRF settings.

Inversely related to depth and frequency.

Aliasing

Reverse wagon wheel effect of racing car is akin to aliasing

Can be reduced by

- Increasing PRF
- Increasing Doppler angle
- Decreasing frequency shift (using a low-frequency Doppler transducer)

Doppler audio signals and spectral waveform varies from vessel-to-vessel and are characteristic of each vessel

Vessel waveform

Central-type arteries (low-resistance vessels) have biphasic spectrum with forward flow during systole and diastole.

Peripheral-type arteries (high-resistance vessels) have triphasic spectrum usually with a sharp systolic peak, a short period of flow reversal in late systole, and near-zero flow in diastole (Figure 31.2).

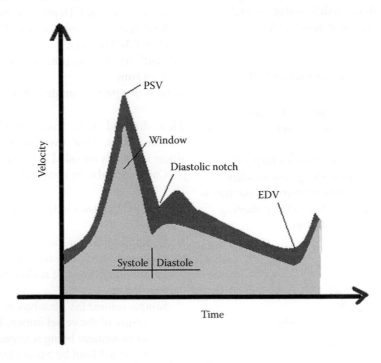

Figure 31.2 Illustrating triphasic spectral waveform of an artery.

32

Obstetric Doppler

One should try to avoid spectral power Doppler during the first trimester because of its certain bio effects.

INTRAUTERINE GROWTH RETARDATION

Definition—Condition in which fetus is not able to achieve its inherent growth potential. Fetal weight <10th percentile for gestational age or abdominal circumference (AC) <2.5 percentile for gestational age.

Etiology

1. Maternal—Diabetes, alcohol, smoking, cardiovascular disease, nutritional deficiencies, anemia, and hypertension
2. Metabolic—Phenylketonuria
3. Infection—CMV, rubella, and herpes
4. Placental—Abruptio, previa, and infarction
5. Genetic—Trisomy 13, 18, 21, Turners syndrome
6. Immunologic
7. Multiple gestations

Types

Symmetrical—Entire body is proportionately small.
    Due to congenital anomaly, genetic disorders, and congenital infections.

Usually diagnosed in the first or early second trimester.
Asymmetrical—Reduced blood supply and nourishment to the fetus usually due to placental insufficiency.
    Usually diagnosed in the third trimester.
    Normal biparietal diameter (BPD), head circumference (HC), and femur length (FL) with AC <2 SD below the mean.
    Associated with reduced AFV.

Indications

1. Forewarning of fetal compromise
2. For placental insufficiency

Stages in ultrasonography prediction for intrauterine growth retardation

1. Evaluate GA in the first trimester—by measuring CRL
    Second trimester—HC, BPD, and AC
    Third trimester—HC, BPD, FL, and AC
2. Assess fetal weight
3. Estimate amniotic fluid index (AFI)
4. Placental grading
5. AC growth <1 centimeter/2 weeks is crucial prognosticator

If parameters are incongruous with the menstrual age, remeasure to check the accuracy. Rescan after—2–4 weeks.

Look for biophysical profile score (BPS)—Normal is 10/10.

Fetal breathing—Two
Fetal movements—Two
Fetal tone—Two
Nonstress test (NST)—Two
AFI—Two
Uteroplacental circuit—Uterine artery, arcuate artery
Fetoplacental circuit—Umbilical artery, middle cerebral artery (MCA), and fetal aorta

Uteroplacental flow is the more important determinant of fetal growth. Abnormal flow in vessels warrants the need of caesarean section

Uterine artery—Branch of internal iliac artery.
Imaging should be done lateral to the uterus where it crosses over the external iliac vessels.
Physiological notch seen in early diastole (s/o high vascular resistance) noted in first half of pregnancy. Persistence of notch beyond 25 weeks is associated with high risk of preeclampsia, PIH, intrauterine growth retardation (IUGR), and placental abruption (Figures 32.1 and 32.2).
Second intrasystolic notch is accompanied by postsystolic notch reflecting extremely high impedance in significant placental insufficiency.

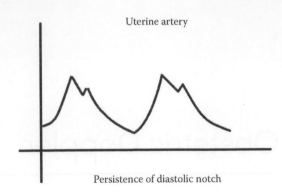

Uterine artery

Persistence of diastolic notch

Figure 32.2 Illustrating abnormal uterine artery waveform after 24 weeks.

Umbilical artery—Diastolic flow cannot be detected in the first 10 weeks due to incomplete villous maturation and can be detected by ~15 weeks with the progression of pregnancy. Reduction in diastolic flow is associated with IUGR (high placental resistance) (Figures 32.3 and 32.4).
Class 0—PI <+2SD—Continuous forward diastolic flow
Class 1—PI >+2SD—Continuous forward diastolic flow
Class 2—Reduction in the diastolic flow

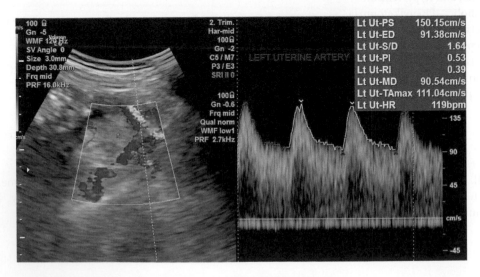

Figure 32.1 Showing normal uterine artery waveform after 24 weeks.

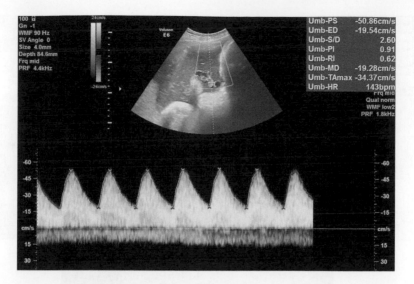

Figure 32.3 Illustrating umbilical artery normal spectral waveform.

Umbilical artery

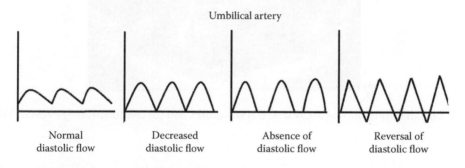

| Normal diastolic flow | Decreased diastolic flow | Absence of diastolic flow | Reversal of diastolic flow |

Figure 32.4 Illustrating spectral waveform of normal and abnormal umbilical artery.

Class 3—Absence of diastolic flow
Class 4—Reversal of diastolic flow
Normal RI—0.65–0.75
Normal PI—1.00–1.26
Middle cerebral artery—Best seen in sylvian fissure as a continuation of intracranial carotid siphon. Conveys 40% of the volume flow from the circle of Willis to each cerebral hemisphere (Figure 32.5).
Normally, MCA has high peak systolic velocity (PSV) and low end diastolic volume (EDV).

In IUGR, diastolic flow increases in MCA due to redistribution of available blood from abdominal and peripheral vessels to the brain. On repeated examination, diastolic flow is completely lost in MCA due to loss of fetal adaptation (Figure 32.6).

Diastolic flow in MCA < Diastolic flow in umbilical artery
Thus, RI (MCA) > RI (Placenta)
Cerobroplacental ratio (CPR)—RI (MCA)/RI (placenta) >1 in normal pregnancy

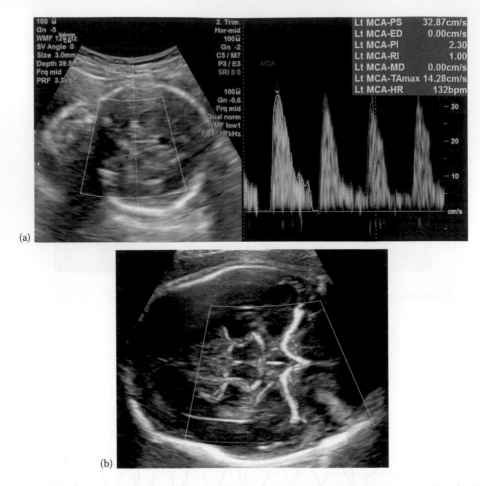

Figure 32.5 **(a)** Illustrating normal MCA spectral waveform and **(b)** Demonstrating circle of Willis.

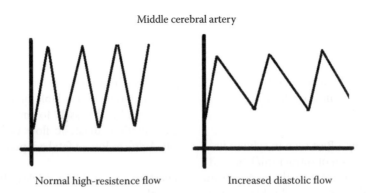

Figure 32.6 Illustrating MCA spectral waveform.

Carotid Doppler

33

Indications

1. H/o atherosclerosis, cardiovascular, cerebro-vascular, or peripheral vascular diseases
2. Aortoarteritis
3. Transient ischemic attacks (TIAs)
4. Subclavian steal syndrome
5. Presence of neck bruit/pulsatile mass

Preparation

Patient in supine position with head extended and turned to the opposite side. No tight clothing.

Anatomy

Three branches of aortic arch:

1. Brachiocephalic trunk
   —Right common carotid artery
   —Right subclavian artery
   —Right vertebral artery
2. Left common carotid artery
3. Left subclavian artery—Left vertebral artery

Common carotid artery bifurcates into internal and external carotid artery at carotid bulb, which is usually 5 centimeters below the angle of mandible.

Internal carotid artery (ICA) is larger than the external carotid artery (ECA). Superior thyroid artery arises from ECA; helps in differentiating ICA from ECA.

Variations in anatomy may occur.

PROTOCOL

Scanning plane—Longitudinal, transverse, and oblique.
Start with B mode.
Study all the vessels—CCA, ICA, ECA, and VA.

Evaluate

1. *Vessel wall* (smooth and regular).
2. Luminal narrowing due to plaque.
   Characterize plaque, if any. Measure actual and available *diameter* of carotid vessels in transverse plane.

$$\% \text{ stenosis} = 100 \times \left(1 - Rd/Nd\right)$$

   Rd—Residual diameter
   Nd—Normal diameter
3. *Carotid intima-medial thickness (CIMT)*—Thickness between lumina—intima and media—adventitia interfaces. Increased thickness is a/w cardiovascular and cerebrovascular pathologies (Figures 33.1 and 33.2).

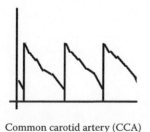
Common carotid artery (CCA)

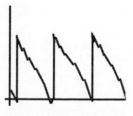
External carotid artery (ECA)

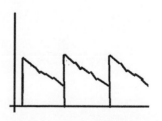
Internal carotid artery (ICA)

Figure 33.1 Illustrating normal waveform in carotid vessels.

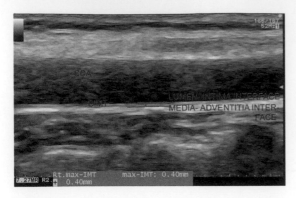

Figure 33.2 Depicts normal carotid intima-medial thickness.

4. Characterize *plaque morphology*
   Hypoechoic—lipid content.
   Echogenicity increases with a rise in collagen content.
   Complex heterogeneous plaque with calcific deposits. Ulcerated plaques have high chances of thromboembolism.
5. Flow characteristics
   In cases of stenosis

Proximal to stenosis—increase in resistance of flow—reduced diastolic flow
At and distal to stenosis—turbulence—broadening of spectral waveform—high velocity

Vessel waveform

ICA—Sharp systolic peak with gradual slope in late systole
   Good forward diastolic flow with diastolic waveform not touching the baseline
   PSV <125 centimeters per second
ECA—Sharp systolic peak
   Minimal/absent flow in diastole
CCA—Combination of ICA and ECA (Figure 33.3)

VERTEBRAL ARTERY

Vertebral artery—arises from first part of subclavian artery.
Usually asymmetric bilaterally with dominant circulation showing high velocity waveform.
Normal vertebral artery shows PSV up to 60 centimeters per second and low-resistance waveform.

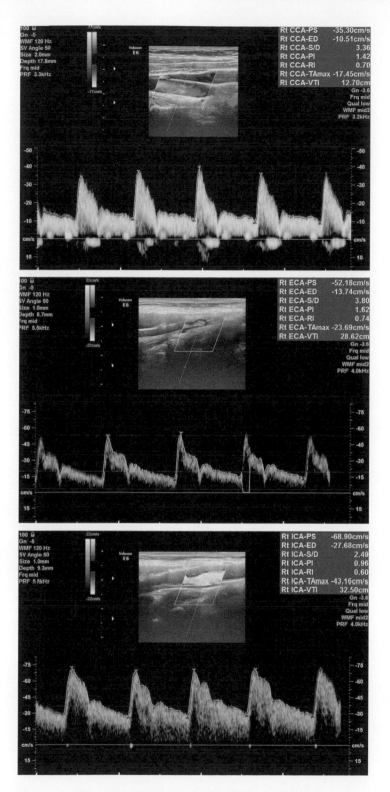

Figure 33.3 Illustrates normal flow and waveform in CCA, ECA, and ICA.

34

Doppler in Portal Hypertension

Normal portal vein (PV) diameter—9–13 millimeters

Normal PV length—6–8 centimeters (splenic vein [SV] + superior mesenteric vein [SMV]) at L1, L2 level

Normal PV pressure—6–10 millimeters of mercury (mm Hg)

Normal PV velocity—12–18 centimeters per second

Normal PV blood flow—500–800 milliliters per minute

Normal flow is Hepatopetal (Figure 34.1)

PV transports blood from GIT to the liver

Etiology

1. Presinusoidal—Extrahepatic—PV thrombosis, compression of PV, and SV occlusion
   Intrahepatic—Malignant infiltration, periportal fibrosis, and toxins
2. Sinusoidal—Cirrhosis
3. Postsinusoidal—Intrahepatic—Cirrhosis
   Extrahepatic—Hepatic vein obstruction (BCS)
   Tumor thrombus/stenosis of IVC
   Most common causes—Extrahepatic portal vein obstruction (EHPO)—45%–50%
   Noncirrhotic portal fibrosis (NCPF)—25%–30%
   Cirrhosis—25%

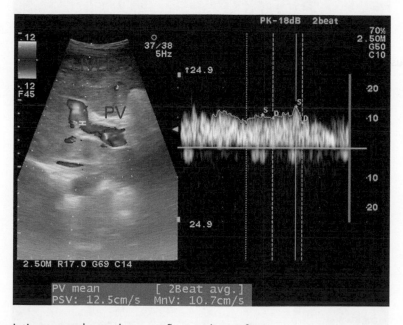

Figure 34.1 Depicting normal portal venous flow and waveform.

Criteria of portal hypertension

1. Increase in PV size >13 millimeters
2. Increase in portal pressure >11 millimeters Hg
3. Loss of normal respiratory/phasic variation in diameter of PV, SMV
4. HepatoFUGAL flow
5. Dilated and tortuous SMV, SV, and HA
6. Recanalization of paraumbilical vein (Figure 34.2)
7. Cavernous transformation—Multiple small vessels at the porta
8. Collateral formation—Paraumbilical (caput medusae), epigastric, splenorenal, hemorrhoidal, paraesophageal, and gastroesophageal
9. Low PV flow velocity <10 centimeters per second (low spectral trace)
10. Splenomegaly
11. Flow may be—Monophasic—Antegrade/retrograde
    Biphasic—Retrograde during inspiration, antegrade during expiration
12. Presence of thrombus—Acute (anechoic, may be overlooked without Doppler) and chronic (hyperechoic) (Figure 34.3)

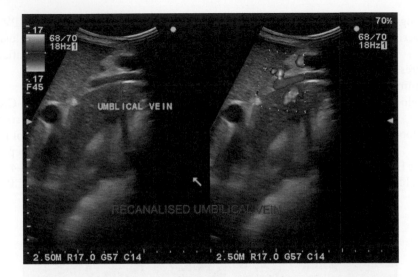

Figure 34.2 Illustrating recanalized umbilical vein.

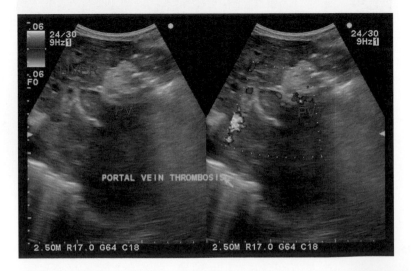

Figure 34.3 Demonstrating portal venous thrombosis.

BUDD CHIARI SYNDROME

Rare disease due to occlusion of hepatic veins or IVC.

Primary—Due to webs in IVC/HVs
Secondary—Due to tumors
Abdominal pain, hepatomegaly, and dilated superficial abdominal vein

B mode—Thrombus in HVs/IVC
   Enlarged caudate lobe
   Ascites, hepatomegaly, and altered regional echogenicity
CDUS—Flow in IVC/hepatic veins changes from phasic to absent, reversed, continuous, or turbulent.
Multiple collaterals in liver.
Chronic BCS—Leads to cirrhosis and PHT.

35

Renal Doppler

Indicated in patients with suspected secondary hypertension to rule out renal artery stenosis (RAS).

CAUSES OF RENAL ARTERY STENOSIS

Atherosclerosis—Proximal vessel involvement

Fibromuscular dysplasia (FMD)—Distal vessel involvement; young females

Arteritis, Takayasu's disease

Aneurysm

Neurofibromatosis

Normal renal arteries arise anterolaterally from the branch of aorta.

Right renal artery arises at 10 o'clock position; passes posterior to IVC.

Left renal artery arises at 4 o'clock position; passes posterior to left renal vein.

B-mode—Comment on kidney size and parenchymal echotexture.

CDUS Scanning—Supine position to trace the origin of renal vessel.

Vessel size is sampled at the origin, hilum, and intrarenally (segmental/interlobar vessels).

Normal waveform

Rapid sharp upstroke in systole. Low-resistance waveform with continuous flow throughout.

Normal PSV—50–160 centimeters per second (<100 centimeters per second).

Normal RI—<0.7 (0.7–1.0 is normal in children <5 years age) (Figure 35.1).

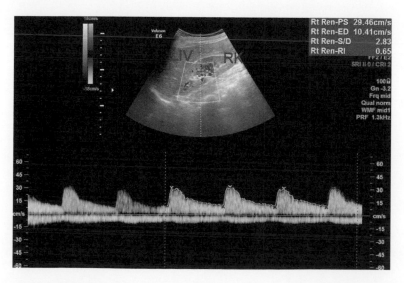

Figure 35.1 Illustrating normal renal artery flow and waveform.

Abnormal measurements

High PSV >180 centimeters per second
(>100 centimeters per second).
High RI >0.7 is s/o obstructive uropathy.
RAR—Renal aortic ratio >3.5 is s/o significant
hemodynamic stenosis >60%.
AT—Acceleration time—Length of time
(in seconds) from the onset of systole to
the peak systole.
>0.07 second is s/o RAS.

Parvus tardus waveform

Parvus (reduced) and tardus (delayed).
Slow systolic upstroke with reduced amplitude
(Figure 35.2).
Pitfalls—Accessory renal artery may be missed.
Angiography is the gold standard to diagnose RAS.
Medical—PTA—Percutaneous transluminal
Angioplasty
Bypass graft
Surgical repair

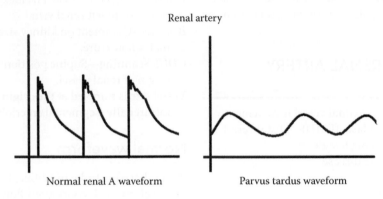

Renal artery

Normal renal A waveform   Parvus tardus waveform

Figure 35.2 Illustrating parvus tardus pattern of waveform.

36

Peripheral Vessel Doppler

ARTERIAL DUPLEX EXAMINATION

Arterial anatomy

Abdominal aorta and its branches.

1. Celiac artery—L_1 level.
2. Superior mesenteric artery—1 centimeter below celiac axis.
3. Renal arteries—Bilateral.
4. Inferior mesenteric artery.
5. Middle sacral artery.
6. Lumbar arteries—Minor branches.
7. Aorta bifurcates into two common iliac arteries, which further branches into external and internal arteries bilaterally.
   External iliac branches into inferior epigastric and the deep circumflex iliac artery continues as the femoral artery.
   Branches of femoral artery—Common femoral artery gives profunda femoris branch and continues as superficial femoral artery, which further continues as the popliteal artery.

Popliteal artery branches:

- Anterior tibial artery becomes dorsalis pedis artery of foot.
- Posterior tibial artery.
- Peroneal artery.

Technique

Patient should be scanned in the supine position for aorta, iliac, femoral, distal tibial vessels, and in prone position for popliteal, proximal, and midtibial vessels.
All the vessels should be studied properly.

B-mode—Normally, the vessel wall is regular and the lumen is anechoic. No thrombus plaque or luminal narrowing is seen.

Normal Doppler spectrum of peripheral vessels—Triphasic pattern.

Sharp systolic peak.

Brief reversal of flow in early diastole and low-frequency forward flow in the late diastole.

Arterial obstruction can be diagnosed by (atheromatous plaques)

1. High velocity in the stenotic zone.
2. Disturbed flow in the poststenotic zone.
3. Collateralization.

Triphasic spectrum becomes monophasic in cases of significant obstruction of 50%–90%.

VENOUS DUPLEX EXAMINATION

Venous anatomy

Superficial system—Long (Great) saphenous and short saphenous veins
Long saphenous vein, seen medially, enters the common femoral vein in the thigh.
Valve is seen at the saphenofemoral junction.
Short saphenous vein, seen laterally, joins the popliteal vein.
Valve seen at the saphenopopliteal junction.
Deep venous system
Paired veins—Anterior tibial veins, posterior tibial veins, and peroneal veins.
Unpaired veins.
Common femoral vein.
Superficial femoral vein.
Popliteal vein.

Perforators—Connects superficial and deep venous system. They have one-way valves, allowing blood flow from superficial to deep.

B-mode—Normal vein has
Thin walls.
Compressible.
Distensible with valsalva.
Anechoic lumen.
Valves may be seen.

Doppler:
Spontaneous flow.
Respiratory phasicity noted.
Augmentation of flow with distal compression.
Absence of retrograde flow on valsalva. Flow ceases during valsalva and increases on its release.

Deep vein thrombosis

B-mode—Distended, noncompressible (normally veins are 100% compressible) veins with luminal echoes.
Nondistensibility of vein with valsalva maneuver (Vein becomes similar to normal artery).

Doppler—Absent/minimal flow with no phasicity and no distal augmentation. Thrombus may get dislodged with distal augmentation, so should not be done.

Varicose Veins
Due to valvular incompetence of saphenofemoral and saphenopopliteal junction.
Dilated superficial veins.
Reflux in superficial veins with the absence of reflux in the deep system.

SUGGESTED READINGS

1. M. Hofer, *Teaching Manual of Colour Duplex Sonography: A Workbook on Colour Duplex Ultrasound and Echocardiography*, Thieme, New York, 2004.

2. P. W. Callen, *Ultrasonography in Obstetrics and Gynecolgy*, 6th ed, Elsevier, Philadelphia, PA, 2016.

3. C. M. Rumack, S. Wilson, J. W. Charboneau, and D. Levine, *Diagnostic Ultrasound: 2-Volume Set*, Elsevier Health US, 2010.

4. S. M. Penny, *Examination Review for Ultrasound: Abdomen & Obstetrics and Gynaecology*, Lippincott Williams & Wilkins, Philadelphia, PA, 2010.

5. W. Herring, *Learning Radiology: Recognizing the Basics*, Mosby Elsevier, Philadelphia, PA, 2007.

6. A. Adam, *Grainger & Allison's Diagnostic Radiology: 2-Volume Set*, Elsevier Health-UK, Kidlington, UK, 2014.

7. D. Sutton, *Textbook of Radiology & Imaging: 2-Volume Set*, Elsevier, New Delhi, India, 2009.

8. S. G. Davies, *Chapman & Nakielny's Aids to Radiological Differential Diagnosis*, Elsevier Health-UK, Kidlington, UK, 2014.

9. W. E. Brant, and C. Helms, *Fundamentals of Diagnostic Radiology: 4-Volume Set*, Wolters Kluwer, Alphen aan den Rijn, the Netherlands, 2012.

10. W. Dahnert, *Radiology Review Manual*, Wolter Kluwer, Alphen aan den Rijn, the Netherlands, 2011.

11. P. E. S. Palmer, B. Breyer, C. A. Brugueraa, H. A. Gharbi, B. B. Goldberg, F. E. H. Tan, M. W. Wachira, and F. S. Weill, *Manual of Diagnostic Ultrasound*, World Health Organisation, Geneva, Switzerland, 1995.

12. World Health Organization (WHO) and World Federation for Ultrasound in Medicine and Biology, *Manual of Diagnostic Ultrasound*, Volume 1 and 2, 2013.

PART V

High-Resolution USG

37

Head and Neck with Thyroid

INTRODUCTION

Anatomy

SALIVARY GLANDS

Normal parotid gland (Figure 37.1) has homogenously hyperechoic echotexture (because of high fat content) in the retromandibular fossa. Small intraparotid lymph nodes are noted. *Stenson's duct* is the main duct. *Retromandibular vein and facial nerve* differentiates between the superficial and deep part of the parotid gland.

Submandibular gland is homogeneous hyperechoic structure at the posterior border of mylohyoid muscle (Figure 37.2). *Wharton's duct* is its main duct. *Facial artery and vein* lie posterior to the gland.

Sublingual gland lies deep to the mylohyoid.

LYMPH NODE LEVELS

Level 1 a—Submental nodes
Level 1 b—Submandibular nodes
    Internal jugular (deep cervical) chain—Levels 2, 3, and 4
Level 2—(Upper cervical) from the base of skull to the hyoid bone
    Around internal jugular vein
Level 3—(Midcervical) from lower border of hyoid to the lower cricoid border
    Lateral to internal jugular vein/common carotid artery
Level 4—(Lower cervical) from cricoid to clavicle
Level 5—Posterior triangle/spinal accessory nodes
Level 6—Anterior to visceral space usually prelaryngeal/pretracheal nodes
Level 7—Superior mediastinal nodes

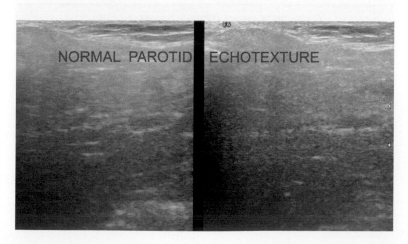

Figure 37.1 Illustrating normal parotid gland echo pattern.

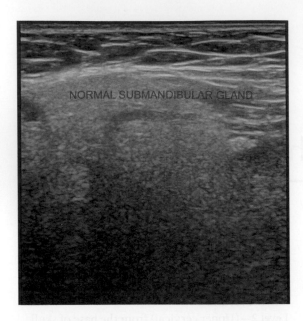

Figure 37.2 Demonstrating normal echo pattern of submandibular gland.

THYROID

Explained in detail in the next paragraph.

PARATHYROID

Usually not visualized routinely due to its small size and deep location.

TECHNIQUE

Supine with neck in extension. Pillow may be placed for the support beneath the shoulder. Both transverse and longitudinal planes are scanned with 7.5–10 MHz linear transducer. Color Doppler and spectral waveform too are helpful.

PATHOLOGY

Lymph nodes

Metastasis in cervical lymph nodes is common in head and neck cancers, lymphoma, inflammatory and infective (tuberculosis) lesions. Evaluation of lymphadenopathy helps in the assessment of prognosis and monitoring response to treatment (Figure 37.3).

Benign nodes
  Usually oval in shape (long axis/short axis
    L/S >1.5–2)
  Iso to hyperechoic in echotexture
  Echogenic hilum is seen suggestive of pre-
    served sinusoidal architecture
  Central hilar flow pattern
Malignant nodes
  Usually round in shape (long axis/short axis
    L/S <2 or 1.5)
  Hypoechoic with pseudocystic/necrotic areas
  Absence of hilum
  Disorganized peripheral flow pattern

Metastatic nodes from papillary thyroid carcinoma may show punctuate calcification.

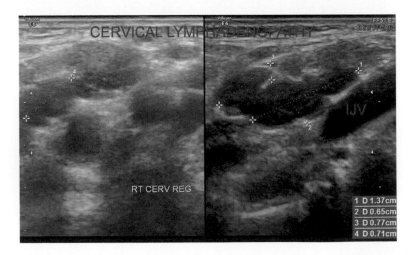

Figure 37.3 Depicting abnormal cervical lymph nodes.

Congenital cystic lesions

BRANCHIAL CLEFT CYSTS

Thin-walled, round/oval anechoic lesion usually seen anterolateral to common carotid artery bifurcation. May show echoes or septae, if infected/hemorrhagic.

THYROGLOSSAL DUCT CYSTS

Thin-walled, round/oval anechoic lesion usually seen anteriorly above the thyroid cartilage in the midline.

LYMPHANGIOMA

Multiseptated, compressible, thin-walled cystic lesion usually located in the posterior triangle of the neck.

RANULA

Thin-walled cystic lesion in the sublingual space; can be imaged both from the skin and transorally with a small probe. Contents become echogenic with thick walls if it gets infected.

If simple ranula extends into the submandibular space, it is known as the plunging ranula.

DERMOIDS/EPIDERMOIDS

Well-defined anechoic lesions (with posterior acoustic enhancement) in the submandibular or sublingual space. It may be homogeneous with low-level echoes or heterogeneous due to presence of fat globules.

Neoplastic lesions

LIPOMA

Well-defined, compressible avascular hypoechoic mass with linear echogenic streaks parallel to the transducer.

NERVE SHEATH TUMORS

Schwannoma and neurofibromas.
Involve vagus nerve, cervical nerve roots, sympathetic chain, and brachial plexus.
Well-defined heterogeneous, hypervascular mass in continuity with the thickened nerve.

SALIVARY GLAND TUMORS

Parotid gland—Pleomorphic adenoma is the most common benign tumor involving the parotid gland.
  Warthin's tumor (adenolymphoma) is the second most common tumor of parotids, usually bilateral with multiple cysts.
  Mucoepidermod carcinoma is the malignant variety.

Infective lesions

Abscesses—Irregular, heterogeneous lesion with necrotic areas and hypervascularity.
Sialedenitis with/without sialoliths.
More common in submandibular gland.
  Inflammation of the gland presenting as enlarged gland with heterogeneous echotexture and high vascularity.
Sialolith (echogenic calculus with acoustic shadowing) sometimes may be seen in the dilated duct.
Acute parotitis
Viral/bacterial
Heterogeneous hypoechoic echotexture of the gland with increased vascularity
Enlarged intraparotid and cervical lymph nodes

HIGH-RESOLUTION SONOGRAPHY OF THYROID GLAND

Introduction

Most sensitive imaging modality available for examination of thyroid gland.
Noninvasive, widely available, inexpensive, and nonionizing.
Real-time USG helps to guide diagnostic and therapeutic interventional procedures.

Ultrasound examination technique

Patient position—Supine with neck hyperextended
Transducer—High-frequency linear array transducer (7–15 MHz)
Plane—Scanning done in the longitudinal and transverse plane

Normal anatomy and sonographic appearance

Thyroid gland consists of two lobes and a bridging isthmus.

Lobe dimensions (Adults)	Longitudinal	40–60 millimeters
	AP	13–18 millimeters

(If AP >20 millimeters with rounding of poles, lobe is said to be enlarged)

Isthmus
    Up to—4–5 millimeters
Volume of thyroid gland (excluding Isthmus)
    10–15 milliliters (females)
    12–18 milliliters (males)

Sonographic Appearance: Thyroid gland appears to be homogeneous in echotexture with medium-level echoes; more than that of the surrounding strap muscles (Figure 37.4).

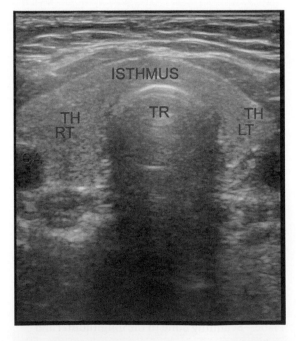

Figure 37.4 Demonstrating normal thyroid gland.

DISEASES OF THYROID GLAND

Incidence—Females > Males
    Nodular thyroid disease is the most common cause of thyroid enlargement.
    Broadly divided into three categories:

1. Diffuse thyroid enlargement
2. Benign thyroid nodule/masses
3. Malignant thyroid nodule/masses

DIFFUSE THYROID DISEASE

Conditions presenting as diffuse enlargement of thyroid gland are as follows:

1. Multinodular goiter
2. Grave's disease
3. Hashimoto's thyroiditis/chronic lymphocytic thyroiditis
4. De quervain's subacute thyroiditis
5. Reidel's thyroiditis

Multinodular goiter

Commonest cause of diffuse asymmetric enlargement of thyroid gland.

Age group—35–50 years, female predilection

USG findings:
    Multiple iso/hyperechoic nodules within diffusely enlarged gland with abnormal intervening parenchyma.
    May undergo degenerative change resulting in varied appearance (Table 37.1).

Table 37.1 Illustrating USG appearances of degenerative changes in multinodular goiter

Degenerative change	Appearance
Cystic	Anechoic
Hemorrhage/Infection	Moving internal echoes/septations
Colloid	Comet tail artifacts
Dystrophic calcification	Coarse/curvilinear echogenic foci

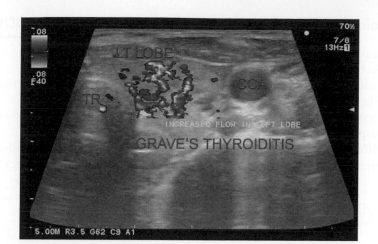

Figure 37.5 Demonstrating Grave's disease.

Grave's disease

Autoimmune disease characterized by thyrotoxicosis

Age group—20–50 years; F > M

USG findings
  Diffusely enlarged thyroid gland, hypoechoic and heterogenous

Color Doppler
  Marked hypervascularity (Figure 37.5)
    Thyroid inferno—Extensive intrathyroid blood flow in both systole and diastole (peak systolic velocity, PSV >70 centimeters per second)

Hashimoto's thyroiditis

Chronic lymphocytic thyroiditis
Autoimmune disorder leading to the destruction of gland and hypothyroidism
Age—>40 years; F > M
Clinically—Painless diffused enlargement of gland
USG findings:
  Focal/diffuse
  Thyroid enlargement with coarse hetero-geneous and hypoechoic parenchymal echopattern
  Multiple discrete hypoechoic micronodules (1–6 millimeters size)
  Fine echogenic fibrous septa—Pseudolobulated appearance
  End stage—Small atrophic gland

Color Doppler findings—Slight to markedly increased vascularity
Associated with increased risk of thyroid malignancy such as follicular/papillary carcinoma and lymphoma
Diagnosis can be confirmed by the pres-ence of serum thyroid antibodies and antithyroglobulin

Dequervain's thyroiditis

Clinical presentation—Painful swelling in the lower neck, fever, and constitutional symptoms typically followed by viral illness.
  Initially thyrotoxicosis followed by hypothyroidism.
USG findings—Enlargement of one or both thyroid lobes with focal hypoechoic map-like areas.
Color Doppler findings—Absence of or decreased blood flow within abnormal areas.

Acute suppurative thyroiditis

Suppurative infection of thyroid gland.

Clinical presentation—Acute onset of fever, pain, asymmetrical swelling of gland (predominantly left sided), and regional lymphadenopathy.
USG findings—Involved lobe appears heteroge-neous and hypoechoic.
  Abscess and cyst formation may occur.

Reidel's thyroiditis

Rare; also known as chronic fibrous thyroiditis, invasive fibrous thyroiditis.

Thyroid gland gradually replaced by fibrous connective tissue; becomes extremely hard.

Encase adjacent vessels/compress/displace or deforms the shape of trachea.

USG findings—Diffusely hypoechoic process with ill-defined margins and marked fibrosis.

THYROID NODULES

Benign
    Adenoma—Follicular and nonfollicular
    Nodular hyperplasia
Malignant
    Carcinoma
    Papillary (75%)
    Follicular (10%)
    Medullary (5%)
    Anaplastic (<5%)
Lymphoma
Metastasis

BENIGN THYROID NODULES

USG features:

1. Iso/hyperechoic with spongiform appearance
2. Width > length
3. Presence of hypoechoic halo around the nodule (complete/uniform)
4. Coarse/curvilinear calcifications
5. Ring down/comet tail artifact (typical of colloid cystic nodule)
6. Perinodular/peripheral flow or spoke-wheel pattern of vessels

Thyroid adenoma

Follicular adenoma more common than nonfollicular

USG appearance—Homogeneous well-defined isoechoic nodule (Figure 37.6).
    Peripheral hypoechoic halo.
Color Doppler findings—Spoke-wheel pattern/peripheral vascularity.

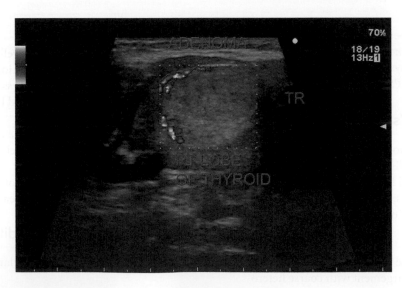

Figure 37.6 Illustrating thyroid adenoma with peripheral vascularity.

MALIGNANT THYROID NODULES

USG features:

1. Microcalcifications (<2 millimeters)
2. Local invasion
3. Lymph node metastases
4. Taller than wider shape
5. Markedly hypoechoic
6. Absence of hypoechoic halo around nodule
7. Ill-defined and irregular margins
8. Solid composition
9. Intranodular central vascularity

Point to note—Multiplicity of nodules is not an indicator of benignity. Incidence of malignancy is the same in solitary as in multiple nodules.

MALIGNANT THYROID MASSES

Risk factors:

1. Age <20 years and >60 years
2. History of neck irradiation
3. Family history of thyroid cancer

Thyroid shield should be used for protection while doing X-ray/CT scan.

Papillary carcinoma

Younger age group; third to fourth decade. Female predilection
USG findings:
   Hypoechogenecity.
   Microcalcifications (punctate hyperechoic foci with or without posterior acoustic shadowing).
   Cervical lymphadenopathy with microcalcifications.
   Lymphatic spread is common; most common cause of cystic lymphadenopathy in the neck.
   Distant metastases rare. Prognosis is good.

Follicular carcinoma

Age group—Fifth decade, female predilection
Blood spread > lymphatic spread
Can be minimally invasive (well encapsulated)/ widely invasive (not well encapsulated)
Distant metastases to bone, brain, and lungs (cannon ball metastases)
USG findings—Irregular margins
   Thick irregular halo
CDUS—Tortuous chaotic internal blood vessels
No USG findings allow for differentiation of follicular carcinoma from adenoma.

Medullary carcinoma

Derived from parafollicular/C cells.
Secretes calcitonin.
Familial—20% cases; component of multiple endocrine neoplasia (MEN) II syndrome. Bilateral and multicentric.
Local invasion and metastases to cervical lymph node more common.
USG findings:
   Hypoechoic mass.
   Bright echogenic foci (calcification) in 80%–90% cases.
   Calcifications more coarse than papillary.

Anaplastic carcinoma

Most aggressive variety
Age group—Elderly
Clinical presentation—Rapidly growing neck mass
USG features:
   Hypoechoic mass with areas of hemorrhage, necrosis, and amorphous calcification.
   Aggressive local invasion; encase and invade blood vessels and neck muscles.
   Worst prognosis.

Thyroid lymphoma

Non-Hodgkin's type of lymphoma.
Age group—Older women. Arises from preexisting Hashimoto's thyroiditis.

Clinical presentation—Rapidly growing neck mass producing symptoms of dysphagia and dyspnea.

USG features—Extremely hypoechoic and lobulated.

CDUS—Neck vessel encasement may be seen.

Metastases

Infrequent.

Main primary tumors spreading to the thyroid gland are malignant melanoma (most common), carcinoma breast, and renal cell carcinoma.

USG features—Solitary/multiple hypoechoic homogeneous masses without calcification.

Thyroid nodules with suspicious USG features are investigated further with FNA biopsy.

38

Breast

INTRODUCTION

Breast is a modified sweat gland.
Functional unit of breast is terminal ductulo lobular unit (TDLU); site of origin of most breast pathologies.

Three zones from superficial to deep (Figure 38.1):

Premammary zone—Subcutaneous zone
Mammary zone—Contains most of the lobar ducts, TDLUs, and fibrous stromal elements of the breast
Retromammary zone—Contains fat, blood vessels, and lymphatics

Echogenicity of structure from superficial to deep:

Hyperechoic—Skin (<2 millimeters thick)
Hypoechoic—Subcutaneous fat (Premammary s/c fat—Lobulated and more hyperechoic than fat elsewhere)
Hyperechoic—Fibroglandular parenchyma (12–20 ducts along with their lobules, fat, and stroma constitutes the breast parenchyma
Hypoechoic—Retromammary fat
Hyperechoic—Muscle (Pectoralis major)

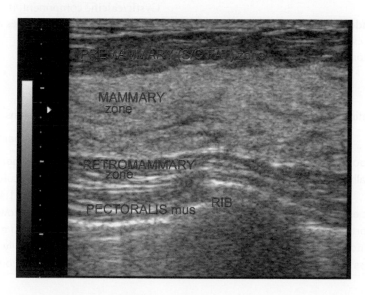

Figure 38.1 Illustrates normal zones of breast.

Echogenicities of various structures:

Hyperechoic structures—Compact interlobular stromal fibrous tissue, anterior and posterior mammary fascia, Cooper's ligament (thin echogenic bands), duct wall, and skin.

Isoechoic—Loose intralobular and periductal stromal fibrous tissue, fat, and epithelial tissues in ducts and lobules.

Hypoechoic—Retromammary fat.

Advantages and indications

1. Ideal in young, pregnant, and lactating females (nonionizing)
2. To differentiate cystic versus solid lesions
3. In tender/inflamed breasts (no compression required as in mammography)
4. To differentiate benign versus malignant lump
5. Follow-up of cysts
6. For lymph nodes
7. As a guide for interventional procedures
8. For implants
9. For clinical breast mass with indeterminate mammogram
10. Follow-up of cancer patients on chemotherapy
11. Suspicious lump in males

Limitations

1. Operator dependent.
2. Low sensitivity especially for microcalcifications.

Technique—Scanning is done in supine and contralateral oblique position with arms comfortably under the head.

ANNOTATION

Side—Right (R) or Left (L)
The clock face with the center at the nipple (1–12 o'clock position)
Zones—Nipple (N), subareolar (SA), axillary (AX), and three circular concentric zones outside the subareolar zone (one, two, and three)
Probe orientation—Radial (RAD), antiradial (ARAD), horizontal, vertical, and oblique planes
Depth of the lesion from the skin

Characteristics to be noted: (Table 38.1)

1. Shape—Round, oval, and its extension along the ducts
2. Size, both in short and long axes, to look for interval changes, if any, on follow-up scans
3. Surface—Smooth, irregular, lobulated, and spiculations
4. Echotexture
   Hypo/iso/hyperechoic
   Homo/heterogeneous
   Cystic/calcific component, if any
5. Fixity to surrounding tissues and underlying muscles
6. Doppler findings

Table 38.1 Illustrating differentiating features of benign and malignant breast lesions

Benign	Malignant
Homogenous, hypo/hyperechoic	Heterogeneously hypoechoic
Well defined, usually smooth margins	Ill-defined, usually spiculated
Wider than tall	Taller than wide (ratio 1:4)
Posterior acoustic enhancement	Posterior acoustic shadowing irregular halo
Architectural distortion less common	Architectural distortion more common
Nipple retraction not seen usually	Nipple retraction usually seen
Skin thickening less common	Skin thickening more common

BENIGN PATHOLOGIES

Normal lactating breast illustrates prominent fluid-filled ducts with echogenic epithelial lining.

Galactocele

Milk-filled cyst results from obstruction of lactiferous ducts; usually located beneath the areola. Resolves spontaneously but aspiration can relieve symptoms.

Fibrocystic disease

Most commonly diagnosed entity in females of reproductive age group

Usually multifocal and bilateral

Patient presents with tender nodular swellings or breast tenderness that worsens during midcycle.

On USG—Patchy areas of echogenicities (prominent fibroglandular tissue) with interspersed hypoechoic/cystic areas without definitive evidence of a mass lesion.

Duct ectasia

Dilated tubular structure (>3 millimeters) filled with fluid or debris (echogenic).

Fibroadenoma

Most common solid benign tumor in the reproductive age group.

It increases in size during adolescence, pregnancy, and lactation. Regresses after menopause.

Smooth, firm, nontender, and may be mobile (mouse within breast).

On USG—Well-defined, ovoid (wider than tall), homogeneous, hypoechoic, and slightly lobulated lesion. May have coarse clumps (popcorn) of calcification. Cystic components may be seen rarely (Figure 38.2).

Cysts

Most common cause of breast lump in ages 35–55 years.

Occurs due to imbalance between secretion and resorption leading to dilatation of lactiferous ducts. Can be single/multiple.

Simple cyst—Well-defined oval to round anechoic lesion surrounded by a thin capsule with a thorough transmission (posterior acoustic enhancement).

Complex cyst—May have septa, echoes, and thick walls.

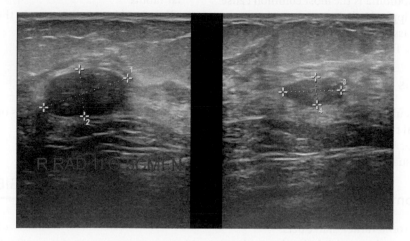

Figure 38.2 Demonstrating fibroadenoma, a benign breast lesion.

Lipoma

Benign, well-defined fat containing lesion compressible on the probe pressure.
USG-Subtle echogenic lesion with thin septations
Surrounded by a thin radio-opaque capsule
May distort the adjacent parenchyma Does not infiltrate/undergo malignant degenera- tion.
May contain calcification (within the areas of fat necrosis)

Intramammary lymph node

Solitary or multiple; usually found in upper outer quadrant
Well-defined, oval, <1 centimeter size and hypoechoic lesion with echogenic hilum
If >1 centimeter, it is suggestive of reaction to inflammatory or metastatic pathology

Hamartoma/fibroadenolipoma

Round, ovoid, and well-circumscribed heterogeneous lesion with peripheral lucent zone. May contain calcification.

Papillomas (Intraductal and intracystic)

Intraductal papilloma is the most common cause of bloody nipple discharge.
Polyploidal mass seen in complex cyst. Difficult to differentiate from carcinoma.

Fat necrosis

Ill-defined spiculated lesion similar to carcinoma with central translucent area. May calcify and may have localized skin thickening.
H/o trauma usually.

Cystosarcoma phylloides

Develops in stroma rather than ducts.
Well-defined, round to oval, lobulated, vascular lesion, often large in size (—6–8 centimeters), and rapidly growing.
Linear anechoic clefts seen in the lesion.

Benign, can recur after excision. Malignant degeneration in <5% cases, can metastasize.

Abscess

Painful breast lesion with high-grade fever and erythema. Complex cystic mass with mobile internal echoes.
May be seen in lactating breasts, tuberculosis, and so on.

Radial scar

Benign.
Spiculated mass with areas of architectural distortion.
Indistinguishable from breast carcinoma on imaging. Excisional biopsy is recommended.

Premature asymmetric ripening

Seen as subareolar mass in prepubertal girls s/o minimal duct development around the nipple.

Gynecomastia

In males, causes uni/bilateral enlargement of breast
May be associated with hyperestrogenism, testicular failure
An ill-defined hypoechoic area in the subareolar region
D/D male breast cancer

Sebaceous cyst

May be anechoic or contain echoes or calcifications.

MALIGNANT PATHOLOGIES

Intraductal carcinoma

Most common type of invasive breast cancer. Spiculated lesion, taller than wide, and heterogeneously hypoechoic lesion with echogenic microcalcifications within (Figure 38.3).

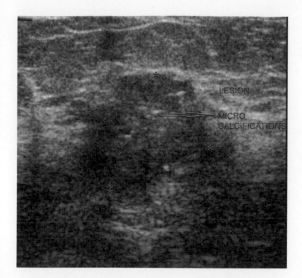

Figure 38.3 An ill-defined, irregular spiculated carcinoma of breast with microcalcifications.

Medullary carcinoma

Usually well defined, younger age group involved in comparison to other carcinomas. Shows rapid growth.

Lobular carcinoma

Usually multicentric and bilateral

Inflammatory carcinoma

Skin thickening, edema, and lymphadenopathy
D/D
Cellulitis
Mastitis

Radiation changes
Locally advanced noninflammatory carcinoma
Edema—Postsurgery/postradiation—Due to venous/lymphatic obstruction—Skin thickening and subcutaneous edema seen

Breast implants

Saline implants are more commonly used in comparison to silicone implants.
Normal intact implant has smooth and thin linear echogenic membrane with anechoic content.

Birads classification

Stage 0—Incomplete assessment. Additional imaging required
Stage 1—Normal on USG with clinical/mammographic abnormalities
Stage 2—Benign, contains intramammary lymph nodes, ectatic ducts, simple cysts, and lipoma
Stage 3—Probably benign—<2% chances of being malignant-simple fibroadenoma, some complex cysts, and papilloma
Stage 4—Suspicious-A—>2% risk of malignancy
Suspicious-B—<90% risk of malignancy
Stage 5—Highly suggestive of malignancy
Stage 6—Biopsy proven

Color Doppler—Increased vascularity seen in certain malignancies.

Elastography, harmonic imaging, and panoramic views provide better characterization.

39

Anterior Abdominal Wall

The anterior abdominal wall is a laminated structure.

ANATOMY

Outer to inner—Skin, superficial fascia, subcutaneous fat, muscle layer, transversalis fascia, and extraperitoneal fat.

Anterior muscle layer—Paired rectus muscle separated in midline by the linea alba. Rectus muscle is enclosed by the rectus sheath.

Anterolateral muscles—External oblique (EO), internal oblique (IO), and transversus abdominis (TA).

HERNIAS

1. *Congenital*—Gastroschisis, Omphalocele (Figure 39.1)
2. *Spigelian*—Lateral abdominal wall—Defect in the aponeurosis of TA muscle

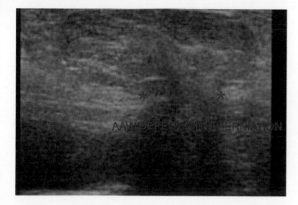

Figure 39.1 Illustrates anterior abdominal hernia.

3. *Lumbar*—Areas of weakness in the flank (lumbar triangles)
   Superior lumbar—Grynfeltt
   Inferior lumbar—Petit
4. *Incisional*—As a complication of abdominal surgery
5. *Inguinal hernia*—Loops of bowel in the inguinal canal
6. *Femoral hernia*—Presents as mass (bowel loop) medial to femoral vein

RECTUS SHEATH HEMATOMA

Posttraumatic, spontaneous (anticoagulant therapy), and bleeding disorder

On USG:

Above the arcuate line—Linea alba prevents the spread of hematoma across the midline. Hence, the hematomas are ovoid on transverse imaging and biconcave on longitudinal imaging.

Below the arcuate line—Blood can spread to the pelvis or cross the midline. It forms a large mass that indents on the dome of the urinary bladder.

FLUID COLLECTIONS

Seroma, liquefying hematoma, abscess (postsurgical/trauma), and urachal cyst (extending from umbilicus to the dome of bladder)

Sterile collections are echo-free in contrast to complicated collections that show septations, layering, and low-level echoes (blood cells/debris)

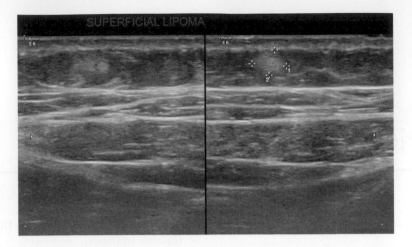

Figure 39.2 Illustrates a small lipoma of AAW.

Neoplasms—Desmoid tumor, lipoma (Figure 39.2), and melanoma metastases

SPLIT IMAGE (GHOST ARTIFACT)

Seen because of the presence of extraperitoneal fat deep to rectus muscle.

In transverse scan plane, sound waves are refracted at the muscle/fat interface in such a way that smaller structures in abdomen/pelvis may be duplicated.

For example—A small gestational sac may appear as two sacs.

One aorta may appear as two aortas.

Scanning the image in longitudinal/oblique plane will resolve the artifact.

Skin (Cellulitis) and Soft Tissue

Cellulitis—Presents with tenderness, skin redness, and warmth.

On USG, appreciated as increased distance between the skin and underlying tissue in comparison to normal unaffected tissue.

Hypoechoic edema in between the subcutaneous tissue layer (cobblestone appearance) (Figure 40.1).

Superficial abscess—Presents with tenderness and fluctuant swelling.

On USG, seen as—Thick, irregularly walled hypo- to heterogeneous collection with moving echogenic particles (debris).

Should be evaluated in two planes and depth from the skin should be marked to guide needle for drainage/aspiration.

Foreign bodies—Certain objects such as glass, wood, metal, and plastic appear echogenic.

Reverberation artifact may be seen.

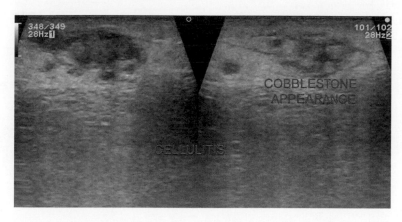

Figure 40.1 Demonstrates cobblestone appearances suggestive of cellulitis.

GIT Sonography

Gas content within the bowel lumen makes the visibility difficult (Table 41.1).

High-frequency linear probe is used.

For identification

Stomach—Gastric rugae
Jejunum—Valvulae conniventes
Large bowel—Haustra

Normal gut is compressible by probe. Abnormally thickened gut is noncompressible.

Graded compression is used in acute appendicitis. Slow-graded compression moves the bowel loops out of the way without any discomfort to the patient.

ACUTE ABDOMEN

1. *Free intraperitoneal gas*—Difficult to detect on USG
   - Echogenic peritoneal stripe
   - Air (ring down artifacts) b/w the abdominal wall and the liver
2. *Loculated fluid collection*—Aperistaltic collection with varying echogenicity

Table 41.1 Illustrating five layers of gut wall (Gut signature)

Mucosa (innermost)	Hyperechoic
Muscularis mucosa	Hypoechoic
Submucosa	Hyperechoic
Muscularis propria	Hypoechoic
Serosa/adventitia	Hyperechoic

3. *Mesenteric lymphadenopathy*—Focal discrete hypoechoic masses of varying size. Loss of echogenic hilum
4. *Edematous bowel loops*
5. *Wall thickening*—Normal gut wall—3 millimeters if distended and 5 millimeters if collapsed
6. *Loss of normal gut signature*

Usually benign lesions involve long segment with concentric thickening and wall layer preservation.

Malignant lesions involve short segment with eccentric disease and wall layer destruction.

ACUTE APPENDICITIS

Normal appendix is compressible with <3 millimeters wall thickness. Graded compression technique (Puylaert) is required.

Presentation—RLQ pain, high WBC count

USG findings
- Blind ended, noncompressible, and aperistaltic tube with diameter >6 millimeters arising from the base of cecum
- Inflamed perienteric fat
- Pericecal collections
- Appendicolith
- Hyperemia of wall

Appendiceal perforation may occur leading to loculated periceal collection, loss of wall layers (Figure 41.1).

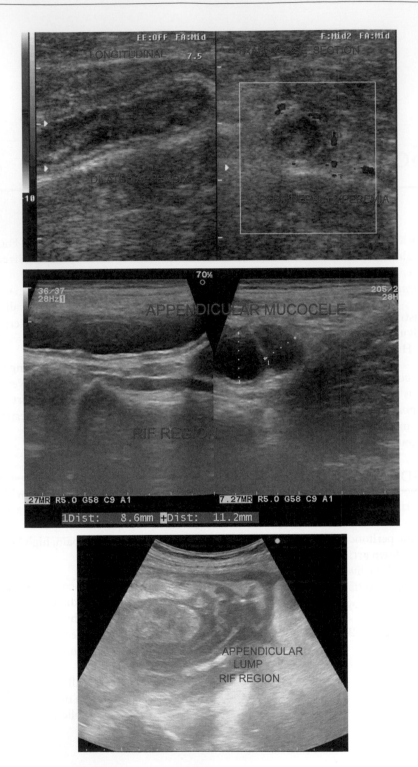

Figure 41.1 Varying presentations of appendicular lesions—appendicitis, mucocele, and appendicular lump.

Mucocele of appendix—Large hypoechoic well-defined RLQ cystic lesion with variable internal echoes.

Sometimes appendix is visualized in the true pelvis (in a suprapubic scan), usually in females due to more capacious pelvis and presents like pelvic inflammatory disease (PID).

D/D

Acute terminal ileitis with mesenteric adenitis
Acute diverticulitis
Acute typhilitis
Acute PID
Ruptured ovarian cyst
Crohn's disease

SMALL BOWEL OBSTRUCTION

Functional (Paralytic ileus)—Hypo/aperistaltic dilated bowel loops (both small and large bowel) (Figure 41.2). Commonly noted in postoperative cases. May occur due to uremia, hypokalemia, and patients on anticholinergic drugs.

Mechanical—Dilatation of intestinal tract proximal to the site of luminal occlusion.

Etiology

Obstruction—Blocking the lumen—Foreign bodies (FBs), ascariasis (Figure 41.3) Bezoars, large gallstones, polypoid tumors, and intussusception.

Intrinsic gut wall abnormalities, strictures leading to luminal narrowing.

Extrinsic bowel lesions, including adhesions.

Postoperative adhesions are the most common cause of small bowel obstruction.

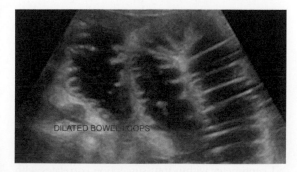

Figure 41.2 Illustrating dilated small bowel loops.

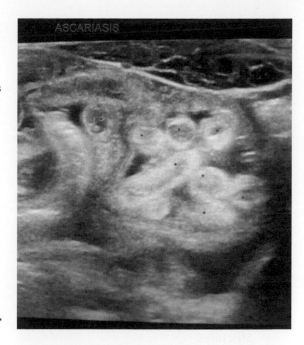

Figure 41.3 Demonstrates multiple ascariasis in the intestinal lumen leading to bowel obstruction.

GASTROINTESTINAL NEOPLASMS

Adenocarcinoma—Most common malignant tumor of the gastrointestinal tract (GIT).

Very common in gastric (prepyloric, antrum, and lesser curvature) and colorectal region.

On USG

- Concentric symmetrical/asymmetrical wall thickening
- Target/pseudokidney sign
- Air in mucosal ulcerations seen as linear echogenic foci with ring down artifacts
- May produce gut obstruction with dilatation, hyperperistalsis proximal to the tumor site
- Usually hypoechoic
- Always look for regional lymphadenopathy and liver metastases

Gastrointestinal stromal tumors (GIST)—Usually found in the stomach and the small bowel. Large exophytic lesions of varying size and echogenicity with central cystic areas due to hemorrhage or necrosis.

Lymphoma—Can be nodular or polypoid
Ulcerative pattern
Infiltrating pattern

Invades adjacent mesentery and lymph nodes

Metastases

Small submucosal nodules or large infiltrative tumors with ulcerations

Ascites, omental thickening, peritoneal nodules, and plaques engulfing/involving the gut loops

INFLAMMATORY BOWEL DISEASE

Crohn's disease

Transmural, granulomatous inflammatory process affecting all the layers of the gut wall. Most commonly involves terminal ileum and colon.

On USG:

- Concentric gut-wall thickening with skip areas.
- Strictures.
- Mucosal abnormalities.
- Creeping fat—Uniformly echogenic halo around the mesenteric border of the gut.
- Lymphadenopathy—Round hypoechoic masses circumferentially surrounding the gut.
- Hyperemia—Complications such as inflammatory mass (abscess), obstruction, fistulae, perianal inflammatory problems, and perforation can be diagnosed.

PEDIATRIC SECTION

Hypertrophic pyloric stenosis

Common in male infants between the 1st week to 3 months of age.

Presents with nonbilious projectile vomiting, olive-shaped palpable mass in epigastrium.

On USG:

- Increased pyloric muscle thickness >3 millimeters.
- Elongated pyloric canal >15 millimeters.
- *Doughnut sign*—Thickened muscle mass may be seen as a hypoechoic layer just surrounding the central echogenic mucosal layer of the pyloric canal.
- Diminished passage of fluid from the stomach into the duodenum.

- Excessive antral peristalsis and reduced peristalsis through pylorus.

Pitfalls

Anisotropic effect—Hypertrophied muscle appears echogenic rather than hypoechoic when imaged in a midlongitudinal plane. Usually occurs at 6 o'clock and 12 o'clock position of the muscle, where the ultrasound beam is perpendicular to the muscle fibers.

Inadequate distension of the gastric antrum may lead to false appearance of thickened muscle layer. Keep the infant in the right posterior oblique position to distend the antrum fully.

Pylorospasm and minimal muscular hypertrophy. Pyloric muscle will be mildly thickened, <3 millimeters.

It may accompany milk allergy or other forms of gastritis.

May resolve spontaneously or may progress to HPS.

INTUSSUSCEPTION

Most common cause of small bowel obstruction in children aged between 6 months and 4 years.

Clinically—Palpable abdominal mass, crampy intermittent abdominal pain, vomiting, and currant jelly stools.

On USG (Figure 41.4):

- Pseudokidney—Oval hypoechoic mass with bright central echoes on longitudinal scan.
- Doughnut/target sign—Similar configuration on transverse scanning.
- Hypoechoic rim represents the edematous wall of the intusussceptum.
- Central echogenicity represents compressed mesentery, mucosa, and intestinal contents.
- Multiple layers and concentric rings.
- Small amounts of peritoneal fluid.
- Lead points such as polyps, lymph nodes, and so on may be seen.
- Large amount of fluid suggests perforation.

CDUS—To identify bowel ischemia.

Peripheral rim thickness >1 centimeter, larger amounts of internal trapped fluid, lymph nodes >1 centimeter within intussusception correlates with decreased success of enema reduction.

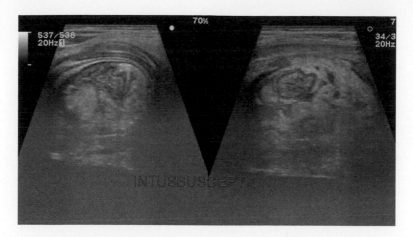

Figure 41.4 Illustrates intussusception.

Management
Air reduction
USG-guided hydrostatic reduction

Transient small bowel intussusception is a frequent occurrence especially in patients with hyperperistalsis. Such intussusceptions are not associated with significant edema in the intussuscepted loops, and hence peripheral rim appears thinner and more echogenic. Spontaneous reduction is observed.

MESENTERIC ADENITIS

RLQ pain
Mesenteric lymph node inflammation. Clusters of tender, enlarged mesenteric lymph nodes >5 in number
Normal appendix
May be associated with mild mucosal thickening in the distal ileum
Self-limiting; associated with viral infections

42

Scrotum

NORMAL ANATOMY AND SONOGRAPHIC APPEARANCE

Testis

Symmetrical ovoid structure; homogeneous echotexture (Figure 42.1).

Length—3–5 centimeters; width 2–4 centimeters; anteroposterior (AP) diameter 3 centimeters.

Surrounded by dense white fibrous capsule (Tunica albuginea).

Epididymis

Elongated crescent-shaped structure.

Length—6–7 centimeters; has head, body, and tail.

Located superolaterally over posterior aspect of testis, iso/hypoechoic relative to testicle.

Tunica vaginalis

Parietal layer → Lines the scrotal wall.

Visceral layer → Envelopes the testis, epididymis, and proximal spermatic cord. Covers the entire testis except small area posteriorly called mediastinum testis (where spermatic cord and its contents join the testicle and seen as a linear echogenic band).

Blood supply

Arterial

- Testicular artery
- Deferential artery
- Cremasteric artery

Venous

Pampiniform plexus—Testicular vein drains into the inferior vena cava (IVC) on the right side and left renal vein on the left side.

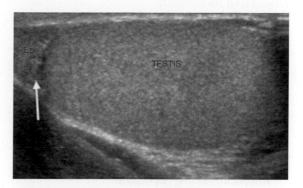

Figure 42.1 Normal scrotal echotexture.

Spermatic cord: Heterogeneous structure (echogenic) in close proximity to the head of epididymis. Color Doppler shows the presence of vessels in it.

USG TECHNIQUE

Supine position with patient's scrotum supported by towels/sheet.

High frequency (7.5–15 MHz) linear array transducer used.

Scanning—Transverse and sagittal planes.

Valsalva maneuver—For evaluation of varicocele.

Indications for Scrotal USG

1. Evaluation of acute scrotal disorder—Torsion, Inflammation, and trauma
2. Evaluation of scrotal fluid collection
   - Hydrocele
   - Pyocele/Hematocele

3. Evaluation of scrotal mass
   - Extratesticular
   - Intratesticular
4. Evaluation of metastatic disease
   - Retroperitoneal lymphadenopathy
   - Testicular involvement—Lymphoma, leukemia
5. Evaluation of varicocele in infertile men
6. Evaluation of undescended testis

BENIGN CONDITIONS

Discovered incidentally

Cyst of Tunica albuginea—Mean age 40 years.
   Usually solitary and unilocular
Cyst of Tunica vaginalis—Rare; anechoic ±
   septations. Echoes d/t. Hemorrhage may
   be seen
Intratesticular cyst—Simple, well-defined cyst
   with posterior acoustic enhancement

1. Tubular ectasia of rete testis:
   Idiopathic, benign condition
   Partial/complete obstruction of efferent duct-
      ules leading to cystic dilation
   B/L and asymmetrical
   USG findings:
   Peripheral elongated structure containing
      multiple small cystic structures. No
      calcification, no solid component, and no
      flow on color Doppler.
2. Epidermoid cysts
   Benign, well circumscribed.
   Second to fourth decade.
   USG findings:
   Alternating rings of hyperechogenicity
      and hypoechogenicity leading to
      characteristic ONION RING SIGN
      (Whorled appearance)
   No flow on Doppler imaging (c.f. testicular
      masses)
3. Abscess—Complication of epididymo-orchitis
   usually
   Infectious causes → Mumps, small pox, influ-
      enza, and typhoid.
   Noninfectious → Testicular torsion, infected
      tumor
   USG findings:
   Enlarged testicle containing cystic mass with
      hypoechoic/mixed echogenic areas

4. Scrotal tuberculosis:
   On USG:
   Enlarged hypoechoic, heterogeneous epididy-
      mis with or without calcifications.
   Testicular involvement from epididymal
      extension.
   Enlarged hypoechoic testis with nodular
      appearance.
5. Scrotal sarcoid: Rare; irregular hypoechoic
   solid masses in testes/epididymis.
6. Adrenal rests
   In patients with congenital adrenal
      hyperplasia.
   USG—B/L hypoechoic, peripherally located
      with spoke-like vascularity on Doppler.
7. Scrotal calcification
   Testicular—Microlithiasis, sarcoid, and
      tuberculosis
   Extratesticular—Scrotal pearls, schistosomiasis
   >5, punctate, nonshadowing, and intratesticu-
      lar calcifications are premalignant.
8. Hydrocele, hemotocele, and pyocele
   Hydrocele—Abnormal accumulation of
      serous fluid between the layers of tunica
      vaginalis
   Congenital—Due to patent processus vaginalis.
   Acquired—Idiopathic, torsion, and tumor.
   USG—Anechoic collection surrounding the
      testis with low-to-medium level echoes due
      to fibrin or cholesterol crystals.
   Hematocele—Due to trauma, surgery, neo-
      plasm, and torsion.
   Pyocele—Due to rupture of abscess.
   USG—Contain internal septations and
      loculations.
9. Varicocele—Abnormally dilated, tortuous, and
   elongated veins of pampiniform plexus poste-
   rior to testis.
   Idiopathic—Due to incompetent valves in
      internal spermatic vein.
   Secondary—Extrinsic pressure due to any
      other lesion and nutcracker syndrome (left
      renal vein compression between aorta and
      superior mesenteric artery).
   More common on the left side as left testicular
      vein drains into the left renal vein.
   USG findings:
   Multiple serpentine anechoic structures
      >2 millimeters in diameter; >1millimeters
      reflux on valsalva (Figure 42.2)
   Associated with infertility.

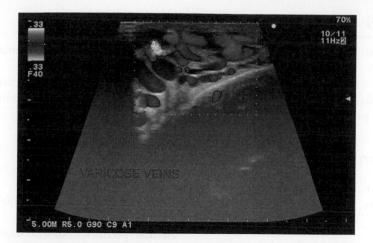

Figure 42.2 Demonstrates varicose veins.

10. *Scrotal hernia*—Presence of bowel loops within scrotum (Valvulae conniventes/haustra) with or without omentum.
11. *Spermatocele*—Due to painless dilatation of epididymal tubules similar to epididymal cyst.
    USG—Anechoic, circumscribed with no/few internal echoes.
    Location—Head of epididymis (c.f. epididymal cyst arise throughout the length of epididymis).

TESTICULAR MALIGNANCY

Germ cell tumors

1. Seminoma—Most common testicular tumor in adults.
   Most common tumor type in cryptorchid testes.
   High risk of seminoma in an undescended testis; also in contralateral normally located tests.
   USG findings:
   Homogeneous hypoechoic echotexture with uniform, low-level echoes without calcification.
   Less aggressive, confined within tunica albuginea.
   Chemo and radiosensitive; favorable prognosis.
   Lymphatic spread is common.
2. *Nonseminomatous germ cell tumors (GCT)*:
   Younger patients' second and third decade.
   More aggressive, invades tunica albuginea.
   More heterogeneous than seminoma with coarse calcifications, areas of hemorrhage/necrosis.
   Frequently cause visceral metastasis.

a. *Mixed GCT*:
   Most common nonseminomatous GCT.
   Second most common testicular malignancy.
   Most common combination—Teratoma and embryonal cell carcinoma.
b. *Pure embryonal cell carcinoma*:
   Younger patients
   Infantile form—Endodermal sinus/yolk sac tumor, common in <2 years
   High alpha-fetoprotein levels
c. *Teratoma*—Contains derivatives of different germinal layers (ectoderm, mesoderm, and endoderm) Can be mature/immature.
   USG—Well defined, markedly heterogeneous with solid/cystic areas.
   Dense echogenic due to calcification/cartilage and so on.
d. *Pure choriocarcinoma*
   Second and third decade.
   Highly malignant.
   Metastasis by hematogeneous and lymphatic routes.
   High β-hcg.

Gonadal stromal tumors:

1. *Leydig cell tumor*: Testicular enlargement and gynecomastia
   USG—Small, solid hypoechoic with peripheral flow on Doppler
2. *Sertoli cell*: Often B/L and multifocal

METASTASES

Lymphoma—Mostly non hodgkin's lymphoma (NHL).

Leukemia.

Nonlymphomatous—Lung and prostate are the most common primaries.

Acute scrotum

Clinical condition characterized by pain, swelling, redness of scrotum, and acute in onset.

Causes of acute scrotal pain

1. Testicular torsion
2. Testicular inflammation (Epididymo-orchitis)
3. Testicular trauma
4. Strangulated hernia
5. Testicular vasculitis and infarction

Testicular torsion

Rotation of testis on the longitudinal axis of spermatic cord.

Pathogenesis

1. Blocked venous drainage (edema and hemorrhage)
2. Impaired arterial flow (Ischemia and hemorrhagic necrosis)

Surgical emergency, delay in intervention can lead to irreversible damage.

Types	More common
Intravaginal	Boys around puberty; 12–18 years
	An anomalous suspension of testis by long stalk of spermatic cord (*Bell clapper* deformity)
Extravaginal	Rare
	Neonates
	Testis and gubernaculum not fixed and freely rotate in the scrotum

USG findings

4–6 hours after onset—Testis enlarged and hypoechoic.

24 hours after onset—Heterogeneous echotexture due to congestion and hemorrhage.

Color doppler

Highly sensitive and specific.

Absent intratesticular blood flow on the affected side.

Twisted spermatic cord with *whirlpool* pattern.

TESTICULAR INFLAMMATION

Most common cause of acute scrotal pain in post pubertal adults.

Cause—*E. coli*, gonococcus, Chlamydia.

Age—40–50 years.

Presents with pain, scrotal swelling, fever, and dysuria.

USG—Enlarged, hypoechoic testis with coarsened echotexture

Reactive hydrocele

CDUS—Increased blood flow

Fournier's gangrene

Necrotizing fasciitis

Seen in diabetics, immunocompromised patients

Cause: Klebsiella, Streprococcus.

Testicular trauma

Direct/straddle injury

Pathology → USG findings:

1. Testicular rupture → Irregularities in testicular contour; heterogeneous echotexture of testis
2. Intratesticular hematoma → Sharply defined hypoechoic lesion

Acute—Blood in tunica vaginalis sac with internal echoes

Chronic—Thick septa, wall thickening
3. Hematocele

CDUS → Disruption of tunica vaginalis with loss of blood supply to the testis.

CRYPTORCHIDISM

One of the most common genitourinary abnormalities in male infant.

Location—Anywhere along the descent pathway from retroperitoneum to scrotum

At or below the level of inguinal canal.

- Localization of undescended testis is important to prevent complications of infertility and cancer.

USG—Undescended testis is smaller and less echogenic than contralateral normally descended testis.

MRI—More sensitive to detect undescended testis in retroperitoneum.

43

Miscellaneous

B SCAN (OPHTHALMIC SONOGRAPHY)

Usually done by high-frequency probes up to 10 MHz. Recently, high-resolution B-scan probes of 20–50 MHz have been manufactured for detailed anatomic resolution of the anterior segment (Figure 43.1).

Done for imaging various ocular and orbital pathologies.

Main method is mainly *contact method* in which the probe is placed directly on the closed eyelid after applying gel. Patient's eye is deviated to

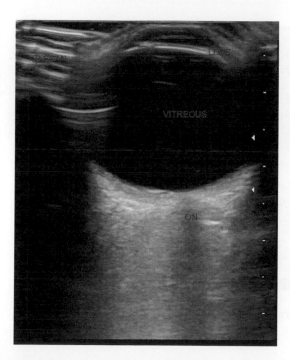

Figure 43.1 Normal B scan illustrating normal anatomy.

right, left, and all directions of gaze to observe the motion of intraocular structures.

Transverse position of the probe delineates the lateral extent of the pathology and longitudinal position determines its radial extent.

Doppler should be used for added information.

Anatomy

Lens—Bright, highly reflective
Membranes (sclera, choroid, and retina)—Highly reflective
Vitreous—Anechoic
Optic nerve—Wedge-shaped hypoechoic in retro-bulbar region
Extra ocular muscles—Hypoechoic

Inferior rectus is the thinnest and superior rectus—Levator palpebrae superior is the thickest. Inferior oblique is usually not visualized except in pathological conditions.

Both the eyes should be examined for comparison.

Indications

Retinal, choroidal, and vitreous detachment
Vitreous hemorrhage
Foreign bodies
Staphyloma and coloboma
Cysticercosis
Asteroid hyalinosis
Lens dislocation
Trauma
Tumors (metastasis, choroidal melanoma and osteoma, hemangioma, retinoblastoma, and orbital tumors) and to look for its extension

TRANSFONTANELLAR SONOGRAPHY

Ideally, a 5–8 MHz vector probe is used, transvaginal probe also provides excellent details. High-frequency linear array may be required for superficial structures. Axial, transtemporal images are assessed with curvilinear probes.

Anterior fontanellar approach is used. Scanning is started and normal anatomy is documented, both in coronal plane (from anterior to posterior) and sagittal and parasagittal (midline, left, and right) planes (Figure 43.2).

Indications

Premature and preterm infants
Germinal matrix hemorrhage
Periventricular leukomalacia (PVL)
Hydrocephalus
Trauma
Suspected mass
Congenital abnormalities
Infections

SUGGESTED READINGS

1. M. Hofer, *Teaching Manual of Colour Duplex Sonography: A Workbook on Colour Duplex Ultrasound and Echocardiography*, Thieme, Stuttgart, Germany, 2004.
2. P. W. Callen, *Ultrasonography in Obstetrics and Gynecolgy*, 6th ed, Elsevier, Philadelphia, PA, 2016.
3. C. M. Rumack, S. Wilson, J. W. Charboneau, and D. Levine, *Diagnostic Ultrasound: 2-Volume Set*, 4th ed., Elsevier Health-US, Philadelphia, 2010.
4. W. Herring, *Learning Radiology: Recognizing the Basics*, Mosby Elsevier, Philadelphia, PA, 2007.
5. A. Adam, *Grainger & Allison's Diagnostic Radiology: 2-Volume Set*, Elsevier Health-UK, 2014.
6. C. M. Rumack and S. R. Wilson, *Diagnostic Ultrasound: Paediatrics, Elsevier, Health UK.*
7. D. Sutton, *Textbook of Radiology & Imaging: 2-Volume Set*, Elsevier, New Delhi, India, 2009.

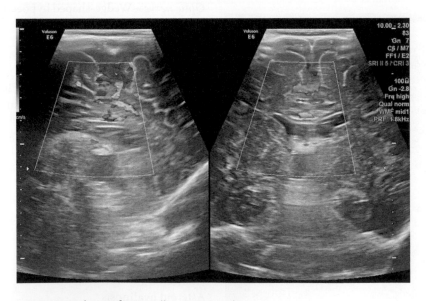

Figure 43.2 Depicts normal transfontanellar sonography.

8. S. G. Davies, *Chapman & Nakielny's Aids to Radiological Differential Diagnosis*, Elsevier Health-UK, 2014.

9. W. E. Brant, and C. Helms, *Fundamentals of Diagnostic Radiology: 4-Volume Set*, Wolters Kluwer, Alphen aan den Rijn, the Netherlands, 2012.

10. W. Dahnert, *Radiology Review Manual*, Wolter Kluwer, Alphen aan den Rijn, the Netherlands, 2011.

11. P. E. S. Palmer, B. Breyer, C. A. Brugueraa, H. A. Gharbi, B. B. Goldberg, F. E. H. Tan, M. W. Wachira, and F. S. Weill, *Manual of Diagnostic Ultrasound*, World Health Organisation, Geneva, Switzerland, 1995.

12. World Health Organization (WHO) and World Federation for Ultrasound in Medicine and Biology, *Manual of Diagnostic Ultrasound*, Volume 1 and 2, H. Lutz, E. Buscarini, Geneva, Switzerland, 2013.

PART VI

USG-Guided Interventions

44

USG-Guided Interventions

1. Thoracocentesis—Chest tap—Pleural effusion tapping
2. Paracentesis—Ascitic fluid tap
3. Cyst aspiration
4. Percutaneous abscess drainage
5. FNAC/Biopsy—Breast, liver, kidney, lymph node, and any peripheral superficial structure
6. Vascular access
7. Suprapubic catheterization

ADVANTAGES

Real-time needle placement
Angled approach (different planes) possible
Color Doppler identifies and avoids the vascular structures in the path
Nonionizing
Minimally invasive with less morbidity
Readily available, relatively inexpensive, and portable
Less time-consuming

DISADVANTAGES

Not suitable for deeper, retroperitoneal structures
Hindrance by the bowel gas
Difficult access in obese patients

PREPROCEDURAL EVALUATION

Coagulation profile should be checked.
Informed written consent.
Prior USG to choose the short possible route, avoiding the adjacent crucial structures.

POSTPROCEDURAL EVALUATION

Monitor patient's vitals
Reimaging for proper procedure

THORACOCENTESIS

Both diagnostic and therapeutic
Done in sitting or lateral decubitus position with the affected side up
Transducer should be perpendicular to the chest
Marker on the probe should point toward the head
Identify diaphragm, liver, spleen, and lung
Locate the largest pocket of fluid and mark it
Note the distance from the transducer to the pleural fluid

PARACENTESIS

Distance from the skin to the fluid. Identify the largest pocket preventing injury to bowel, omentum, and vessels
Distance to the midpoint of collection

CYST ASPIRATION

Patient lies supine or slightly turned to one side.
Arm placed under the head comfortably.
Under aseptic precautions and topical anesthesia, a small needle (seen as white echogenic line on USG) is advanced into the cyst under the guidance of USG. Suction is applied by the syringe to draw fluid out and the lesion collapses.

PERCUTANEOUS ABSCESS DRAINAGE

Done for appendicular, diverticular, amoebic, pyogenic, tubo-ovarian, postsurgical abscesses, and so on (Figure 44.1).

Diagnostic needle aspiration is done.

Single stage—Catheter (8F/12F) is advanced directly into the lesion under the guidance of USG.

Multistage—Done by modified Seldinger technique using a catheter, needle, and guide wire.

Catheter is secured and attached to a drainage bag. Drain should be flushed before removing the catheter.

USG-GUIDED FNA/BIOPSY

Breast lesions:
Focal masses/cysts.
Microcalcifications.
Architectural distortion.
For breast biopsy, try to maintain an angle parallel to the chest wall to reduce the risk of injury to deeper structures.
Liver:
Focal lesions
Diffuse parenchymal disease such as hepatitis B and C, cirrhosis, hemochromatosis, and abnormal liver function tests

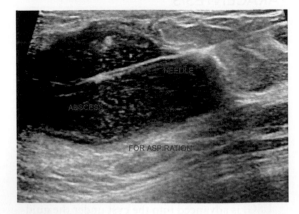

Figure 44.1 Illustrates abscess drainage through a needle.

Ensure that no major vessel, dilated biliary channels, or gallbladder are in the path of needle biopsy

Performed with breath hold in expiration to minimize the risk of injury to the lung or pleura

Kidney
Solid/cystic focal lesions
Nonfocal—Nephropathy/renal transplant rejection
Done in the prone position
Usually taken from lower pole in nonfocal cases
Care should be taken to spare the collecting system and renal hilum to prevent injury to vessels and ureter
Thyroid—Benign versus malignant

COMPLICATIONS

Hemorrhage
Pneumothorax
Bile leakage
Peritonitis
Infection
Needle track seeding
Minor complications such as vasovagal reaction, transient hematuria, and self-limiting resolving pneumothorax

USG-GUIDED VASCULAR ACCESS

Under proper aseptic conditions, using color Doppler, identify and differentiate between artery and vein.

On B mode, veins have thin and compressible walls, nonpulsatile, and expand with the valsalva. Too much pressure on the vein leads to collapse of the vein.

Internal jugular vein—Lies anterolateral to internal carotid artery (Central venous cannulation)

Femoral vein—Lies medial to femoral artery.

USG-guided cannulation is advantageous in patients with dehydration, scarring on skin, and patients with history of difficult access.

SUPRAPUBIC CATHETERIZATION

Required in patients with acute urinary retention where urethral catheterization is difficult or contraindicated.

LUMBAR PUNCTURE

Use to identify spinous processes of lumbar vertebrae (Echogenic with acoustic shadowing) and delineate interspinous space for needle entry.

TRANSJUGULAR INTRAHEPATIC PORTOSYSTEMIC SHUNTS

Usually done for relief of symptomatic portal hypertension, refractory ascites.

Right hepatic vein via infrahepatic IVC is accessed through the transjugular route.

Puncture needle is passed from the hepatic vein to the intrahepatic portal vein and a shunt is created.

The tract is dilated to ~10 millimeters with monitoring of portal pressure gradient.

Bridging stent is left in place.

Complications such as stent occlusion and stenosis, hepatic vein stenosis may occur.

PART VII

Recent Advances in Sonography

45

Recent Advances in Sonography

3D USG

Works similar to traditional 2D USG except that ultrasound waves are directed from multiple angles. These waves are reflected back and captured and provide enough information to construct a 3D image.

Advantages

1. Multiplanar
2. High-spatial resolution
3. Less scan time
4. Reproducibility
5. Images can be stored for revaluation
6. Teleconsultation
7. Postprocessing (Tomographic ultrasound imaging [TUI], volume rendering (VR), and automatic slicing)
8. Measurement of volume and vascularity of the lesion

Acquisition

1. Manual (Mechanical scanner)—Probe is moved by the user during data acquisition.
2. Sensor based (Sensed free-hand technique). Transmitter generates pulsed electromagnetic field, which is detected by the sensor attached to the transducer.
3. Automatic (Free-hand scanning without position sensing).
   Anatomy is acquired as a dataset.
   Each anatomical scan plane can be rotated on *XYZ*-axis to get high-quality image.

Indications

Gynecologic—
  Congenital uterine malformation.
  Characterization of adnexal masses.
  Infiltration of adjacent organs.
  Volume measurement.

Obstetric (Figure 45.1)—Fetal face, cleft lip, and palate, nuchal thickness, cardiac, skeleton and neural tube defects, and so on.

Saline sonohysterography
Prostate
Tumors
For interventions

Augmenting capabilities for data storage allows extended field of view (EFOV), panoramic imaging.
  3D + Time—4D (3D motion video—real-time video of anatomy)
  Fast sequences of 3D images are processed real time through 30 frames per second volumetric imaging.
  Utilizes the similar frequency of sound waves akin to normal USG, but the sound waves are directed from many more angles.
  3D + Time + Sound—5D

Accelerated focused US imaging

Permits high-speed 3D imaging of dynamic structures such as cardiac valves

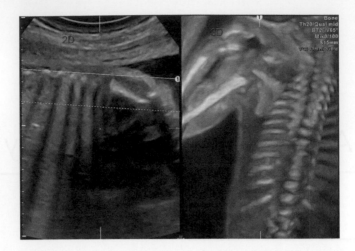

Figure 45.1 Illustrating 2D and 3D USG of fetus for comparison.

Equivalent to parallel MRI
High-spatial resolution (increased number of lines/images)
Sharpening of image

TUI—Tomographic ultrasound imaging, volume USG

Exhibits multiple parallel slices within a volume of dataset similar to CT and MRI.
Displaying multiple slices at 1 time → expeditious and easier viewing of volume information.
Minimizes scan time.

VCI–C—Volume contrast imaging–coronal

Only 4D real-time technique that exhibits *coronal* plane imaging.
Enhanced tissue contrast resolution.
Based on 4D volumetric data acquisition, a volume-rendering process performed on a thick slice of tissue data.
Provides scan planes, not accessible by conventional B-mode scanning.
Facilitates detection of suspicious lesions.

APPLICATIONS

- Obstetrics imaging—If fetal position obscures anatomy in 2D scan.
- Gynecologic—Enables the user to exactly position a scan plane along the axis of the uterus.

- Urology—Evaluating incontinence.
- Breast—Aids in differentiating benign versus malignant nodules by depicting architecture of lesion and adjacent breast parenchyma.

SRI—Speckle reduction imaging

Speckle is an intrinsic artifact in an USG image that obscures the underlying anatomy and deteriorates the spatial and contrast resolution.
First real-time algorithm that contributes to remarkable reduction in the speckle.
Enhances edges and borders.
High SNR.

STIC—Spatial temporal imaging correlation

Evaluates complex anatomical relationships
Acquires 4D USG at rates of >40 volumes per second
Advantageous adjunct to fetal echocardiography (since fetal heart beats very rapidly)

MR/USG-GUIDED HIGH INTENSITY FOCUSED ULTRASOUND (HIFU) ABLATION

Principle

Basic principle is identical to using a magnifying glass to focus sunlight and generate heat for burning.

Absorption of ultrasound energy in the tissue during transmission induces cavitation damage and coagulative thermal necrosis.

Therapeutic and minimally invasive method to direct acoustic energy into the body using an acoustic lens to concentrate multiple intersecting beams of ultrasound specifically on a target in the body.

Indications

Uterine fibroids and adenomyosis
Tumors, both primary and metastatic, even at difficult locations (liver, prostate, breast, pancreas, and soft tissue sarcomas)

Advantages

Minimally invasive
Less painful
Safe to ablate tumors in the vicinity of major blood vessels where surgical resection may prove disastrous as the blood flow dissipates the thermal energy from the vessel wall
Expeditious recovery
No remaining scars
Cost-effective

Virtual CT sonography

System for synchronizing multiplanar reconstructed CT scans with corresponding conventional USG images in real time
For detection of small hepatic nodules
Allow bed-side percutaneous USG-guided biopsy

Contrast enhanced (Gas-filled microbubbles)

Right sided (R to L shunts).
Left sided.
Microbubbles increase reflectivity of blood by nonlinear back scatter.
Two forms:
Untargeted—Echocardiography
Targeted—Disease/organ specific
For monitoring response to therapy

TRANSPERINEAL ULTRASOUND

Technique

2D—Linear array, convex linear (transvaginal probe)
3D—Hybrid probe (volume rendered)
Scan planes—Sagittal, coronal, and axial
Cover with glove; place transducer on perineum and apply minimal pressure

Three compartments:

Anterior—Bladder, urethra
Middle—Vagina, uterus
Posterior—Rectum, anus

Advantages

1. Nonionizing
2. Inexpensive
3. Enables better understanding of dynamics and potential treatment of pelvic floor disorders
4. Easier on patient, examiner
5. Can visualize tensionless vaginal tapes, slings, and mesh

Limitations:

1. Multicompartment disease
2. Operator dependency
3. Limited FOV
4. Equipment variation
5. Rectocele, rectal intussusception, and perineal hypermobility cannot be differentiated

Applications

1. *Stress urinary incontinence*
   Evaluates bladder neck mobility
   USG findings:
   Funneling of internal urethral meatus on valsalva or at rest
   Rectovesical angle >120 degrees on valsalva (normal b/w 90–120)
   Bladder neck descent >3 millimeters (distance from bladder neck to symphysis pubis) on valsalva
2. *Pelvic organ prolapse*
   Movement of pelvic organs below reference line (Inferior aspect of symphysis)
   Cystocele—Abnormal bladder descent

Enterocele—Posterior to vagina
Rectocele—Bulging of rectal wall at anorectal
 junction
3. *Fecal incontinence*—Thinning/disruption of
 internal/external anal sphincter
4. Postoperative assessment of prolapse, incontinence, and surgical complications
5. 3D transperineal affords dynamic depiction of
 tensionless vaginal tape (TVT)
6. Cervical length measurement during the third
 trimester as an alternative to transvaginal
 sonography (TVS)

INTRAVASCULAR ULTRA SOUND

Introduction—Valuable adjunct to angiography
providing new insights into diagnosis and treatment of coronary disease.
 Equipment

1. Catheter—Incorporating a miniaturized
 transducer
2. Console—Containing the electronics necessary
 to reconstruct the image
3. High-frequency 20–50 MHz transducer—For
 excellent resolution

Applications

1. Gold standard for *in vivo* plaques
 Allows tomographic assessment of the
 • Lumen area
 • Plaque size
 Distribution and composition of plaque
2. For vessels that are problematic to image by
 angiography
 Diffusely diseased segments
 Ostial/bifurcation stenosis
 Eccentric plaques
 Angiographically foreshortened vessel
3. Provides unique images of the atherosclerotic
 plaque not merely the lumen.
 Lipid laden—Echolucent, homogeneous
 Fibromuscular—Low intensity (soft echoes)
 Fibro/calcified—Echogenic
  Fibrous—Less bright but more than muscle/
   fat tissue.
  Calcified—More echogenic.

ELASTOGRAPHY

Introduction

Elasticity of soft tissue depends on

1. Their molecular building blocks
 (fat, collagen).
2. Micro- and macroscopic structural organization of these blocks.

The standard medical practice of soft tissue palpation is based on the qualitative assessment of the
stiffness of tissue.

Principle

Stiffness/strain of soft tissue is used to detect/
classifying tumor. A tumor or suspicious cancerous growth is 5–28 times stiffer than back-
ground of normal soft tissue (Figure 45.2).
 When a mechanical compression/vibration
is applied, the tumor deforms less than the surrounding tissue, that is, strain is less in tumor.
 This new technology allows hardness/stiffness
of biological tissues to be estimated and imaged.
 Certain malignant tumors manifest them-
selves as change in mechanical properties of
tissue.
 *USG acoustic radiation force impulse imaging
(ARFII)*—Uses acoustic radiation force to generate images of mechanical properties of soft
tissue.

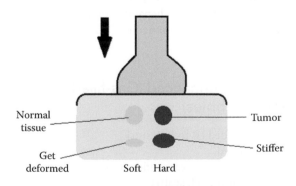

Figure 45.2 Illustrating elastography principle.

Applications

1. Liver fibrosis quantification.
2. To assess elasticity in nonalcoholic fatty liver disease.
3. In the normal breast, glandular structures (firmer) > connective tissue > subcutaneous fat.
4. Colorectal cancer—Images layered structure. Guides treatment decision.
   Preoperative tumor/lymph node staging.
5. Prostate—For targeting biopsies (Figure 45.3).

TISSUE HARMONIC IMAGING

Introduction

Amplitude of harmonic signal is significantly lower than the fundamental frequency band (Figure 45.4).

Harmonics arise only after a beam has reached a certain depth in tissue to avoid noise and scattering.

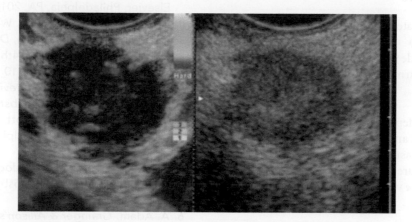

Figure 45.3 Elastography imaging depicting cancerous tissue.

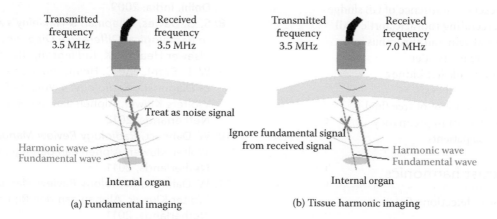

Figure 45.4 Depicting principles of **(a)** Fundamental Imaging and **(b)** Tissue harmonic imaging.

Principle

In conventional USG, same frequency spectrum that is transmitted into the patient is subsequently received to produce the sonographic image.

In tissue harmonic imaging (THI), higher harmonic frequencies generated by nonlinear wave propagation of USG beam through tissues are used to produce the sonogram.

Second harmonic or twice the fundamental frequency is used for imaging.

Advantages

1. Improved lateral resolution (reduced width of USG beam)
2. Reduced side lobe and body wall artifacts (because harmonic signal is generated within tissue)
3. High SNR
4. Improved depiction of finely detailed anatomy
5. Both cystic and solid lesions
6. High contrast and spatial resolution
7. Any structure that is fluid filled/obscured by haze may be visualized with greater clarity and sharpness

Applications

1. Fatty liver
2. Metastasis in liver
3. Presence or absence of GB sludge
4. Descending thoracic aortic wall
5. Portal vein and thrombus in it
6. Pancreatic border
7. Lower pole left kidney
8. Small renal cysts
9. Small amount of free fluid
10. Fetal heart in pregnancy
11. Obese patients

Contrast harmonics

Improves detection of

1. Deep seated and small vessels
2. Vessel with low slow flow
3. Abnormal tumor vessels
4. Stenotic lesions
5. Ischemic regions

Harmonic B mode
Harmonic color Doppler
Harmonic spectral Doppler
Harmonic power mode

SUGGESTED READINGS

1. M. Hofer, *Teaching Manual of Colour Duplex Sonography: A Workbook on Colour Duplex Ultrasound and Echocardiography.*
2. P. W. Callen, *Ultrasonography in Obstetrics and Gynecolgy*, 6th ed, Elsevier, Philadelphia, PA, 2016.
3. C. M. Rumack, S. Wilson, J. W. Charboneau, and D. Levine, *Diagnostic Ultrasound: 2-Volume Set*, 4th ed., Elsevier Health-US, Atlanta, GA, 2010.
4. S. M. Penny, *Examination Review for Ultrasound: Abdomen & Obstetrics and Gynaecology*, Lippincott Williams & Wilkins, Philadelphia, PA, 2010.
5. W. Herring, *Learning Radiology: Recognizing the Basics*, Mosby Elsevier, Philadelphia, PA, 2007.
6. A. Adam, *Grainger & Allison's Diagnostic Radiology: 2-Volume Set*, Elsevier Health-UK, Kidlington, UK, 2014.
7. D. Sutton, *Textbook of Radiology & Imaging: 2-Volume Set*, Elsevier, New Delhi, India, 2009.
8. S. G. Davies, *Chapman & Nakielny's Aids to Radiological Differential Diagnosis*, Elsevier Health-UK, Kidlington, UK, 2014.
9. W. E. Brant, and C. Helms, *Fundamentals of Diagnostic Radiology: 4-Volume Set*, Wolters Kluwer, Alphen aan den Rijn, the Netherlands, 2012.
10. W. Dahnert, *Radiology Review Manual*, Wolter Kluwer, Alphen aan den Rijn, the Netherlands, 2011.
11. W. Dahnert, *Radiology Review Manual*, Wolter Kluwer, Alphen aan den Rijn, the Netherlands, 2011.
12. World Health Organization (WHO) and World Federation for Ultrasound in Medicine and Biology, *Manual of Diagnostic Ultrasound*, Volume 1 and 2, 2013.

Sample Questions

WRITE SHORT NOTES ON

Q.1 USG principle.

Q.2 USG transducer.

Q.3 Real-time ultrasound.

Q.4 Piezoelectric effect.

Q.5 Ultrasound gel.

Q.6 Spatial resolution.

Q.7 Time-gain compensation (TGC).

Q.8 Ultrasound artifacts.

Q.9 Biological effects of ultrasound.

Q.10 Chaperone.

Q.11 Segmental anatomy of liver.

Q.12 Vascular anatomy of liver.

Q.13 USG findings in liver cirrhosis with portal hypertension.

Q.14 USG findings in hepatitis.

Q.15 Infective liver lesions.

Q.16 Focal hepatic lesions.

Q.17 Varying ultrasound presentation of liver metastasis.

Q.18 USG findings in acute cholecystitis.

Q.19 Causes of nonvisualization of gallbladder.

Q.20 Causes of thickened gallbladder wall.

Q.21 USG findings in different types of cholangitis.

Q.22 Cholangiocarcinoma.

Q.23 Choledochal cysts classification.

Q.24 Classify various cystic and solid lesions of spleen.

Q.25 Causes of splenomegaly.

Q.26 USG findings in acute pancreatitis along with its complications.

Q.27 Adenocarcinoma of pancreas.

Q.28 Various cystic neoplasms of pancreas.

Q.29 Normal variants of kidney.

Q.30 Congenital anomalies of kidney.

Q.31 Various infective lesions of kidney.

Q.32 Renal cystic disease.

Q.33 Neoplastic lesions of kidney.

Q.34 Medical diseases of genitourinary tract.

Q.35 Renal cell carcinoma.

Q.36 How infant kidney differs from adult kidney.

Q.37 Hydronephrosis.

Q.38 Enumerate branches of aorta.

Q.39 Enumerate tributaries of IVC.

Q.40 Abdominal aortic aneurysm.

Q.41 Difference between prepubertal and postpubertal uterus.

Q.42 Appearance of endometrium during different phases of menstrual cycle.

Q.43 Abnormal uterine bleeding.

Q.44 Menorrhagia.

Q.45 Endometrial polyps.

Q.46 Leiomyomas.

Q.47 Adenomyosis.

Q.48 Pelvic inflammatory disease—USG findings.

Q.49 Cystic lesions of pelvis.

Q.50 Endometriosis.

Q.51 Carcinoma cervix.

Q.52 Classify various ovarian tumors.

Q.53 How will you differentiate benign versus malignant ovarian tumors on ultrasound?

Q.54 Describe zonal anatomy and ultrasound appearance of prostate.

Q.55 Carcinoma prostate.

Q.56 Enlist various retroperitoneal and intraperitoneal organs.

Q.57 Describe various peritoneal cavity spaces.

Q.58 Short note on ascites.

Q.59 FAST.

Q.60 USG in acute abdomen.

Q.61 USG findings in abdominal tuberculosis.

Q.62 USG findings in RIF pain.

Q.63 USG findings in appendicitis.

Q.64 Cystic lesions of liver.

Q.65 Benign lesions of liver.

Q.66 Hepatocellular carcinoma.

Q.67 USG appearance of normal intrauterine gestation in first trimester.

Q.68 Double decidual sac sign.

Q.69 Early pregnancy failure.

Q.70 Complications of first trimester pregnancy.

Q.71 Placental abruption.

Q.72 Placenta previa.

Q.73 Amniotic fluid estimation.

Q.74 Gestational trophoblastic neoplasia.

Q.75 Ectopic pregnancy.

Q.76 Hydrops.

Q.77 Signs of intrauterine fetal death on USG.

Q.78 USG findings of incompetent cervix.

Q.79 Congenital uterine malformations.

Q.80 Pc PNDT Act.

Q.81 Alimentary tract lesions diagnosed *in utero*.

Q.82 Imaging of placenta.

Q.83 Imaging in infertility.

Q.84 Doppler evaluation in IUGR.

Q.85 Transvaginal scan in female infertility.

Q.86 Sonographic features of markers of chromosome abnormality on antenatal ultrasound.

Q.87 Vascular and structural abnormalities of umbilical cord.

Q.88 Describe various sonographic findings in complications of twin pregnancy.

MCQs

Q.1 After ovulation the follicle collapses to form
   (a) Graffian follicle
   (b) Corpus luteum
   (c) Corpus hemorrhagicum
   (d) Corpus albicans

Q.2 hCG (Human Chorionic Gonadotropin) is produced by
   (a) Amniotic sac
   (b) Yolk sac
   (c) Syncytiotrophoblasts
   (d) Decidua

Q.3 In pregnancy, involution of corpus luteum is prevented by
   (a) LH
   (b) FSH
   (c) Both LH and FSH
   (d) hCG

Q.4 The function of yolk sac is
   (a) Transfer of nutrients
   (b) Angiogenesis
   (c) Hematopoesis
   (d) All of the above

Q.5 In amniotic band syndrome all are true except
   (a) Occurs due to developmental chorio-amniotic separation
   (b) May lead to limb body wall complex
   (c) Embryo may extend into the space between amnion and chorion
   (d) Occurs due to iatrogenic rupture of amniotic membrane.

Q.6 All are the components of umbilical cord except
   (a) Umbilical vessels
   (b) Umbilical cord cyst
   (c) Vitelline duct
   (d) Allantois

Q.7 Umbilical artery arises from
   (a) Fetal internal iliac artery
   (b) Fetal external iliac artery
   (c) Maternal internal iliac artery
   (d) Maternal external iliac artery

Q.8 Umbilical artery in newborns become
   (a) Median umbilical ligament
   (b) Medial umbilical ligament
   (c) Ligamentum teres
   (d) Ligamentum venosum

Q.9 Allantois becomes
   (a) Urachus
   (b) Median Umbilical ligament
   (c) Both (a) and (b)
   (d) Medial umbilical liament

Q.10 Acute hemorrhage is usually
   (a) Hyperechoic
   (b) Hypoechoic
   (c) Sonolucent
   (d) None of the above

Q.11 Most common site of implantation in ectopic pregnancy is
   (a) Cornua of endometrial canal
   (b) Intramural portion of tube
   (c) Ovary
   (d) Cervix

Q.12 Drug of choice for medical management of ectopic pregnancy is
   (a) Mifepristone
   (b) Misoprostol
   (c) Methotrexate
   (d) All of the above

Q.13 Definitive diagnosis of ectopic pregnancy is done by
   (a) Transabdominal USG
   (b) Color Doppler
   (c) Transvaginal USG
   (d) Laparoscopy

Q.14 Earliest cystic structure in posterior aspect of embryonic head, which later forms the normal fourth ventricle
(a) Prosencephalon
(b) Rhombencephalon
(c) Mesencephalon
(d) Telencephalon

Q.15 Echogenic structures filling the lateral ventricles of head normally are
(a) Choroid plexus
(b) Choroid angioma
(c) Diencephalon
(d) Debris

Q.16 Normal physiological herniation of anterior abdominal wall is seen up to
(a) 6 weeks
(b) 8 weeks
(c) 12 weeks
(d) 18 weeks

Q.17 Bony defect in the skill with associated protrusion of intracranial contents
(a) Exencephaly
(b) Iniencephaly
(c) Holoprosencephaly
(d) Encephalocele

Q.18 Banana sign is characteristic of
(a) Spina bifida
(b) DWM
(c) Agenesis of corpus callosum
(d) Anencephaly

Q.19 All are associated with trisomy 21 except
(a) Absent nasal bone
(b) Increased nuchal fold thickness
(c) Duodenal atresia
(d) Strawberry head

Q.20 Midline abdominal wall defect is
(a) Omphalocele
(b) Exomphalos
(c) Both a and b
(d) Gastroschisis

Q.21 Normal fetal kidneys appear by around
(a) 6 weeks
(b) 10 weeks
(c) 12 weeks
(d) 16 weeks

Q.22 All are features of trisomy 18 except
(a) Absent nasal bone
(b) Strawberry-shaped skull
(c) Choroid plexus cysts
(d) Cystic hygroma

Q.23 All are soft markers for chromosomal defects except
(a) Choroid plexus cysts
(b) Echogenic bowel
(c) Echogenic intracardiac focus
(d) Hydrops

Q.24 For diagnosing ventriculomegaly measured as transverse measurement of atrium of occipital horn should be
(a) >3 millimeters
(b) 6 millimeters
(c) >10 millimeters
(d) >20 millimeters

Q.25 Enlarged cisterna magna is said if size is
(a) >10 millimeters
(b) >20 millimeters
(c) >5 millimeters
(d) 15 millimeters

Q.26 Lateral, paraumbilical defect of abdominal wall
(a) Omphalocele
(b) Gastroschisis
(c) Exomphalos
(d) Pentalogy of centrall

Q.27 Major source of amniotic fluid after 16 weeks is
(a) Fetal urine
(b) Fetal lungs
(c) Placenta
(d) Fetal skin

Q.28 All are features of B/L renal agenesis except
(a) Severe oligohydramnios
(b) Key-hole sign
(c) *Lying down* adrenal sign
(d) Nonvisualization of kidneys and bladder

Q.29 Gender determination can be done by
(a) 8 weeks
(b) 10 weeks
(c) 12 weeks
(d) 16 weeks

Q.30 Artifact caused by air/gas is known as
(a) Mirror image artifact
(b) Comet tail artifact
(c) Posterior acoustic shadowing
(d) Posterior acoustic enhancement

Q.31 All are retroperitoneal organs except
(a) Aorta
(b) Liver
(c) Kidneys
(d) Duodenum

Q.32   Transitional call carcinoma is commonly found in
(a)   Liver
(b)   Urinary bladder
(c)   Spleen
(d)   Duodenum

Q.33   Wilms tumor is a malignant pediatric mass involving
(a)   Adrenal gland
(b)   Spleen
(c)   Kidneys
(d)   Urinary bladder

Q.34   Which of the following is not considered an intraperitoneal organ?
(a)   Liver
(b)   Spleen
(c)   Gallbladder
(d)   Duodenum

Q.35   All are retroperitoneal organs except
(a)   Adrenal glands
(b)   Uterus
(c)   Ovaries
(d)   Aorta

Q.36   Most common benign tumor of liver is
(a)   Hemangioma
(b)   Hepatic adenoma
(c)   Focal nodular hyperplasia
(d)   Simple liver cyst

Q.37   Pancreatoblastoma is
(a)   Benign tumor of pediatric pancreas
(b)   Malignant tumor of pediatric pancreas
(c)   Benign tumor of adult pancreas
(d)   Malignant tumor of adult pancreas

Q.38   Oncocytoma is a tumor of
(a)   Liver
(b)   Spleen
(c)   Kidneys
(d)   Pancreas

Q.39   A tumor consisting of tissue from all three germ cell layers is
(a)   Angiomyolipoma
(b)   Osteosarcoma
(c)   Osteochondroma
(d)   Teratoma

Q.40   All are structures located at porta hepatis except
(a)   Main portal vein
(b)   Hepatic vein
(c)   Common bile duct
(d)   Hepatic artery

Q.41   Which of the following is the first branch of abdominal aorta as it passes below the diaphragm
(a)   Left gastric artery
(b)   Celiac artery
(c)   Superior mesenteric artery
(d)   Phrenic artery

Q.42   On USG, ligamentum teres lying near to left portal vein appears hyperechoic because of
(a)   Water
(b)   Fat
(c)   Lymph nodes
(d)   Vessel

Q.43   On USG, diffuse thickening of gallbladder with hyperechoic foci and comet tail artifact is seen in
(a)   Carcinoma GB
(b)   Cholecystitis
(c)   Adenomyomatosis
(d)   Polyposis

Q.44   USG shows central dot sign in
(a)   Carolis disease
(b)   Focal nodular hyperplasia
(c)   Cholangitis
(d)   Abscess
(Central dot—Multiple cystic areas with central dot of PV branch surrounded by dilated biliary ducts).

Q.45   To detect gestational sac on TAS, what should be the minimum size?
(a)   5–10 millimeters
(b)   10–17 millimeters
(c)   15–20 millimeters
(d)   20–30 millimeters

Q.46   12 weeks antenatal scan can diagnose which anomaly
(a)   Multicystic dysplastic kidney
(b)   Anencephaly
(c)   Corpus callosum agenesis
(d)   Skeletal dysplasias

Q.47   Strawberry gallbladder is seen in
(a)   Porcelain GB
(b)   Polyposis of GB
(c)   Cholesterolosis
(d)   Carcinoma GB

Q.48   Cyst within cyst sign seen in
(a)   Tuberculosis cavity
(b)   Aspergilloma
(c)   Hydatid cyst
(d)   Amoebic abscess

Q.49 Investigation of choice for detecting minimal ascites
(a) MRI Scan
(b) PET Scan
(c) USG
(d) XR abdomen—Lat decubitus view

Q.50 Bedside screening tool in patients with trauma
(a) Mobile XR scan
(b) USG
(c) Peritoneal lavage
(d) CT scan

Q.51 Small well-defined hyperechoic lesions in liver are s/o
(a) Simple liver cyst
(b) Hepatic adenoma
(c) Hemangioma
(d) Biliary hamartoma

Q.52 B/L small smooth kidneys with raised echogenicity and loss of CMD is seen is
(a) Nephrolithiasis
(b) Medullary cystic ds/Nephronophthisis
(c) Medullary sponge kidney
(d) Multicystic dysplastic kidney

Q.53 All are ionizing except
(a) CT Scan
(b) USG
(c) XR
(d) PET–CT

Q.54 USG probe is made of
(a) Gadolinium
(b) Quartz
(c) Lead zirconate
(d) Strontium

Q.55 Which is echogenic on USG?
(a) Vessels
(b) Bone
(c) Bile
(d) Bladder

Q.56 USG shows enlarged kidneys with raised echogenicity in a child s/o
(a) ADPCKD
(b) ARPCKD
(c) MCDK
(d) Medullary cystic disease

Q.57 Hypertrophied column of Bertin is a
(a) Renal inflammation
(b) Sinus tumor
(c) Normal variant
(d) Uropathy

Q.58 Standard diagnostic criteria for ADPCKD on USG of each kidney
(a) 0–2 cysts
(b) 3–5 cysts
(c) 6–7 cysts
(d) Tiny innumerable cysts

Q.59 Modality of choice for imaging adrenal glands in neonates is
(a) CT scan
(b) USG
(c) MRI
(d) MIBG Scan

Q.60 In BPH, all are seen except
(a) Enlarged lateral lobes of prostate
(b) Residual urine in bladder
(c) Fish hook distal ureter
(d) Trabeculated bladder

Q.61 Most common cause of micronodular cirrhosis is
(a) Alcohol
(b) Chronic viral hepatitis
(c) Both (a) and (b)
(d) None of the above

Q.62 All of these are features of cirrhosis except
(a) Coarse and heterogeneous echotexture
(b) Surface nodularity
(c) Starry sky pattern
(d) Enlarged caudate lobe

Q.63 All of these are features of chronic hepatitis except
(a) Hepatomegaly
(b) Enlarged caudate lobe
(c) Thickened GB wall
(d) Periportal cuffing

Q.64 Most common liver tumor seen in females using OCPs
(a) Focal nodular hyperplasia
(b) Hepatic adenoma
(c) Fibrolamellar carcinoma
(d) Hemangioma

Q.65 All of the following are true for hydatid cyst in liver except
(a) Caused by *Entamoeba histolytica*
(b) Cysts have three layers
(c) Shows water lily sign
(d) Calcification may occur

Q.66 WES sign in GB s/o
(a) Gallstones
(b) GB carcinoma
(c) Perforation of GB
(d) Normal variant

Q.67 All are the tumors of stomach except
(a) Gastrinoma
(b) Gastric lymphoma
(c) Linitis plastica
(d) All of the above

Q.68 Lesser Sac is the space b/w
(a) Liver and kidney
(b) Stomach and pancreas
(c) Spleen and kidney
(d) Liver and spleen

Q.69 Collection of abdominal fluid within the peritoneal cavity a/w neoplasm is
(a) Peritoneal ascites
(b) Exudative ascites
(c) Transudative ascites
(d) Chylous ascites

Q.70 Ultrasound wave are high frequency sound waves over
(a) 2 kHz
(b) 20 kHz
(c) 20 MHz
(d) 20 Hz

Q.71 USG waves are generated by
(a) Generators
(b) Amplifier
(c) Transducer
(d) Transmitters

Q.72 Transducers are
(a) Transmitters of ultrasound
(b) Receivers of ultrasound
(c) Both (a) and (b)
(d) None of the above

Q.73 Real-time image means
(a) Multiple B-mode images in rapid sequence
(b) Multiple A-mode images in rapid sequence
(c) M-mode images
(d) None of the above

Q.74 USG waves propagate as
(a) Transverse waves
(b) Longitudinal waves
(c) Circular motion
(d) All of the above

Q.75 The average propagation speed for soft tissues is
(a) 1,440 meters per second
(b) 340 meters per second
(c) 1,540 meters per second
(d) 4,620 meters per second

Q.76 All are true except
(a) High frequencies are readily absorbed and scattered than lower frequencies.
(b) High frequencies have better resolution but less depth.
(c) Low frequencies penetrate better but have less resolution.
(d) High frequencies penetrate better.

Q.77 All are specular reflectors except
(a) Fetal skull
(b) Walls of vessels
(c) Liver
(d) Diaphragm

Q.78 Linear array transducers are used for
(a) Breast ultrasound
(b) Cardiac ultrasound
(c) Transvaginal ultrasound
(d) Upper abdomen

Q.79 Sector scanner is used for all except
(a) Gynecological examination
(b) Cardiac examination
(c) Upper abdomen
(d) Thyroid

Q.80 Acoustic enhancement is shown by
(a) Clear cyst liquids
(b) Bones
(c) Stones
(d) Ribs

Q.81 True for coupling agent is
(a) Eliminates air between transducer and the surface of patient.
(b) Water is a good coupling agent.
(c) Oil can also be used as a long-term coupling agent.
(d) It forms a barrier between transducer and the skin of the patient.

Q.82 Which of the following is correct?
(a) Borders of portal veins have brighter echoes.
(b) Borders of hepatic veins are bright (reflective walls)
(d) Both portal vein and hepatic veins have bright borders.
(d) None of the above

Q.83 Normal cross-sectional diameter of the adult aorta at the level of xiphoid is
(a) 1 centimeters
(b) 3 centimeters
(c) 4 centimeters
(d) 5 centimeters

Q.84 Invasion of IVC is common in all except
(a) RCC
(b) HCC
(c) Adrenal carcinoma
(d) Splenic carcinoma

Q.85 Hyperechoic structure in the liver
(a) Falciform ligament
(b) Portal vein
(c) Hepatic artery
(d) Common bile duct

Q.86 Which of the following is more echogenic?
(a) Liver
(b) Pancreas
(c) Spleen
(d) Kidneys

Q.87 All are findings of acute hepatitis except
(a) Tender hepatomegaly
(b) Thickened edematous GB
(c) Normal hepatic parenchyma
(d) Multiple echogenic lesions

Q.88 Von Meyenberg complexes are associated with
(a) Liver abscess
(b) Biliary cystadenomas
(c) Biliary hamartomas
(d) Hemangiomas

Q.89 Bulls eye sign is characteristic of
(a) Hydatid cyst
(b) Oncocytoma
(c) Focal nodular hyperplasia
(d) Metastases

Q.90 Normal GB appears distended in all patients except
(a) High fat diet
(b) Low fat diet
(c) On intravenous nutrition
(d) Dehydrated

Q.91 All are causes of mobile echogenic lesions in GB lumen except
(a) Calculi
(b) Polyp
(c) Sludge
(d) Ascariasis

Q.92 All are causes of nonmobile echogenic lesions in GB lumen except
(a) Polyp
(b) Tumor
(c) Sludge
(d) Mucosal fold

Q.93 Normal thickness of GB wall
(a) <3 millimeters
(b) 3–5 millimeters
(c) >5 millimeters
(d) None of the above

Q.94 All are the causes of generalized thickening of GB wall except
(a) Cholecystitis
(b) CHF
(c) Hepatitis
(d) GB polyp

Q.95 Normal CBD diameter in young:
(a) 6–7 millimeters
(b) 10–12 millimeters
(c) 1–2 centimeters
(d) None of the above

Q.96 Portal vein is formed by the confluence of
(a) Hepatic vein and splenic vein
(b) Splenic vein and gastric vein
(c) Hepatic vein and superior mesenteric vein
(d) Splenic vein and superior mesenteric vein

Q.97 Normal splenic vein diameter
(a) Up to 3 millimeters
(b) Up to 10 millimeters
(c) Up to 20 millimeters
(d) None of the above

Q.98 Small, hyperechoic pancreas is suggestive of
(a) Acute pancreatitis
(b) Carcinoma head of pancreas
(c) Chronic pancreatitis
(d) All of the above

Q.99 Hypoechoic, enlarged pancreas is seen in all except
(a) Acute pancreatitis
(b) Chronic pancreatitis
(c) Tumor
(d) Cystic lesion of pancreas

Q.100 Normal diameter of the head of pancreas
(a) ~1 centimeters
(b) ~2 centimeters
(c) ~3 centimeters
(d) ~4 centimeters

Q.101 All are causes of splenomegaly except
(a) Malaria
(b) Infarct
(c) Lymphoma
(d) Portal hypertension

Q.102 Which of the following is most echogenic?
(a) Renal sinus
(b) Renal cortex
(c) Renal medulla
(d) Renal pyramids

Q.103 Renal sinus comprises all except
(a) Fat
(b) Vessels
(c) Collecting system
(d) Pyramids

Q.104 All are causes of shrunken kidney except
(a) Acute renal vein thrombosis
(b) Chronic renal failure
(c) Renal artery stenosis
(d) End-stage renal vein thrombosis

Q.105 All are the causes of localized bladder wall thickening except
(a) Neoplasms
(b) Granuloma
(c) Prostatic obstruction
(d) Trauma

Q.106 Cystic lesion within the bladder near a ureteric orifice is
(a) Cystocele
(b) Ureterocele
(c) Utricle
(d) All of the above

Q.107 Small bladder is seen in
(a) Prostatic enlargement
(b) Urethral stricture
(c) Tuberculosis
(d) Urethral valves

Q.108 The endometrium appears thick hyper-echogenic in
(a) Proliferative phase
(b) Luteal phase
(c) Secretory phase
(d) None of the above

Q.109 Complex ovarian lesion with calcification (bone/teeth) is a characteristic of
(a) Endometriomas
(b) Hemorrhagic cyst
(c) Brenner's tumor
(d) Dermoid cyst

Q.110 Anomaly scan is best done at
(a) 10–12 weeks
(b) 18–20 weeks
(c) 28–30 weeks
(d) 34–36 weeks

Q.111 Double echogenic ring (Double decidual sign) is highly s/o
(a) Choriocarcinoma
(b) Ectopic pregnancy
(c) Normal pregnancy
(d) Incomplete abortion

Q.112 Snow storm effect in uterus is characteristic of
(a) Hydatidiform mole
(b) Ectopic pregnancy
(c) Endometriomas
(d) Myomas

Q.113 Most reliable parameters for estimating gestational age up to 11 weeks
(a) BPD
(b) AC
(c) FL
(d) CRL

Q.114 Widest diameter of skull from side-to-side
(a) BPD
(b) HC
(c) Cephalic index
(d) All of the above

Q.115 Anencephaly can be recognized as early as
(a) 5–6 weeks
(b) 11–12 weeks
(c) 14–15 weeks
(d) 18–20 weeks

Q.116 All of the following are associated with polyhydramnios except
(a) Jejunal obstruction
(b) CNS anomalies
(c) Urinary tract anomaly
(d) Maternal diabetes

Q.117 All of the following are associated with oligohydramnios except
(a) Renal anomalies
(b) Rupture of membranes
(c) Gastrointestinal obstruction
(d) Postmaturity

Q.118 Spalding's sign is characteristic of
(a) Fetal death
(b) Hydrops
(c) Anencephaly
(d) Spina bifida

Q.119 Thickened placenta is seen in all except
(a) Rh incompatibility
(b) Maternal preeclampsia
(c) Abruptio placenta
(d) Moderate maternal diabetes

Q.120 Normal umbilical cord has
(a) Two arteries one vein
(b) Two veins one artery
(c) One artery one vein
(d) Two arteries two veins

Q.121 Which of the following is a side effect of USG?
(a) Ionizing
(b) Invasive
(c) Heating
(d) None of the above

Q.122 Intradecidual sign seen around
(a) 10 weeks MA
(b) 2 weeks MA
(c) 7 weeks MA
(d) 5 weeks MA

Q.123 The first structures to be seen within the gestational sac
(a) Yolk sac
(b) Embryo
(c) Heart
(d) None of the above

Q.124 Double bleb sign represents
(a) Yolk sac and embryo
(b) Amnion and yolk sac
(c) Amnion and vitelline duct
(d) Yolk sac and vitelline duct

Q.125 All of the following should be suspicious for early pregnancy failure except
(a) MSD >8 millimeters no yolk sac on TVS
(b) MSD >16 millimeters no embryo on TVS
(c) CRL >5 millimeters no cardiac activity on TVS
(d) CRL >2 millimeters no cardiac activity on TVS

Q.126 Scan at 11–14 weeks detects all except
(a) Nuchal translucency
(b) Fetal structural defects
(c) Anencephaly
(d) Absence of nasal bone

Q.127 All are criteria for early pregnancy failure except
(a) Distorted GS shape
(b) Thin trophoblastic reaction (<2 millimeters)
(c) Low position of GS within the endometrial cavity
(d) Growth at the rate of 1.1 m/d

Q.128 All are the criteria of embryonic demise except
(a) Visualization of amnion in the absence of embryo
(b) Visualization of amnion in the presence of embryo
(c) Irregularly marginated collapsed amnion
(d) Calcified yolk sac

Q.129 Decidual cast is suggestive of
(a) Hydatidiform mole
(b) Normal pregnancy
(c) Ectopic pregnancy
(d) Fibroids

Q.130 Irregular cranial end with no visible echogenic calvarium suggests
(a) Anencephaly
(b) Encephalocele
(c) Acrania
(d) Hydranencephaly

Q.131 Lemon-shaped head is characteristic of
(a) Corpus callosum agenesis
(b) Spina bifida
(c) Dandy walker malformation
(d) Holoprosencephaly

Q.132 Recurrent second trimester loss is associated with
(a) Chromosomal abnormality
(b) Fetal structural defects
(c) Cervical insufficiency
(d) None of the above

Q.133 Lambda or twin peak sign is s/o
(a) DC/DA
(b) MC/DA pregnancy
(c) MC/MA
(d) Conjoined twins

Q.134 Lobe of Liver between GB fossa and round ligament is
(a) Caudate lobe
(b) Quadrate lobe
(c) Left lobe
(d) Right lobe

Q.135 All are the causes of enlarged heterogeneous uterus except
(a) Endometriomas
(b) Diffuse leiomyoma
(c) Adenomyosis
(d) Endometrial carcinoma

Q.136 The least likely cause of complex cystic adnexal mass with positive HCG except
(a) Ectopic pregnancy
(b) Corpus luteal cyst
(c) Theca lutein cysts
(d) Hemorrhagic cysts

Q.137 Calculus that grows to fill the collecting system is
(a) Jackstone calculus
(b) Staghorn calculus
(c) Cholesterol calculus
(d) Uric acid calculus

Q.138 All are the causes of thick echogenic endometrium except
(a) Normal IUP
(b) Ectopic pregnancy
(c) Retained product of conception
(d) Endometriomas

Q.139 All are causes of elevated maternal serum alpha-fetoprotein (MSAFP) except
(a) Multiple gestation
(b) Neural tube defects
(c) Down syndrome
(d) Fetal demise

Q.140 Cause of diffusely enlarged placenta after second trimester
(a) Maternal hypertension
(b) Toxemia
(c) IUGR
(d) Maternal diabetes

Q.141 Absent stomach bubble in fetus is a/w all except
(a) Esophageal atresia
(b) Ladd's bands
(c) Swallowing abnormality
(d) Oligohydramnios

Q.142 Hyperemesis gravidarum is a/w all except
(a) Obesity
(b) Molar pregnancy
(c) Bacterial gastroenteritis
(d) Multiple pregnancy

Q.143 Complications of fetal macrosomia
(a) Shoulder dystocia
(b) TORCH infections
(c) Pulmonary hypoplasia
(d) Club foot

Q.144 Which of the following is not a branch of celiac artery?
(a) Splenic artery
(b) Gastroduodenal artery
(c) Left gastric artery
(d) Common hepatic artery

Q.145 Arterial supply to GB is via
(a) Celiac artery
(b) Gastroduodenal
(c) Cystic artery
(d) Common hepatic artery

Q.146 IVC is _____ to right renal artery
(a) Posterior
(b) Medial
(c) Lateral
(d) Anterior

Q.147 Which structure crosses b/w aorta and SMA?
(a) Left renal vein
(b) Celiac a
(c) Right renal artery
(d) Left renal artery

Q.148 What regulates flow of bile into the duodenum at the Ampulla of Vater?
(a) Dust of Wirsung
(b) Duct of Santorini
(c) Sphincter of Oddi
(d) Stenson's duct

Q.149 Attenuation in ultrasound increases as distance
(a) Increases
(b) Decreases
(c) Remains same
(d) none of the above

Q.150 Which of the following is not a factor determining spatial resolution?
(a) Wavelength
(b) Acquisition
(c) Pulse length
(d) Transmit intensity

Q.151 Lowest mean propagation velocity is seen in
(a) Water
(b) Blood
(c) Fat
(d) Air

Q.152 Attenuation decrease as frequency
(a) Decreases
(b) Increases
(c) Remains same
(d) None of the above

Q.153 When the length of vessel is halved
  (a) Resistance is halved
  (b) Viscosity is doubled
  (c) Velocity is halved
  (d) Resistance is doubled

Q.154 Narrowest point of USG beam
  (a) Near field
  (b) Focus
  (c) Far field
  (d) Fresnel zone
  (*Hint: Narrowest point with best lateral resolution and highest intensity*)

Q.155 Scanning with low frame rate on USG machine is suggestive of
  (a) Narrow scan area
  (b) Decreased system depth
  (c) Increased system depth
  (d) Small scan area
  (*Hint: Multiple focal zones/increased depth → low frame rate*)

Q.156 If gain is doubled and input power remains same. What will be the output power?
  (a) Halved
  (b) Unchanged
  (c) Doubled
  (d) Four times

Q.157 Ultrasound wave attenuation is denoted by
  (a) kHz
  (b) MHz
  (c) W/cm^2
  (d) Decibels

Q.158 Centre operating frequency in pulsed wave transducers is determined by
  (a) Crystal thickness
  (b) Propagation velocity
  (c) Backing material thickness
  (d) Spatial pulse length

Q.159 Most common age group for seminoma is
  (a) 16–30 years
  (b) 0–5 years
  (c) 35–50 years
  (d) 50–70 years

Q.160 Pulse repetition frequency (PRF) is determined by
  (a) Medium through which the sound travels
  (b) Depth of tissue being examined
  (c) Amplitude of wave
  (d) Total output power

Q.161 Two identical systems produce a pulse, one of 0.7, microseconds and other of 1.6 microseconds. Which will have better temporal resolution?
  (a) 0.7 microseconds
  (b) 1.6 microseconds
  (c) Both have same
  (d) Undetermined
  (*Hint: Pulse duration is not related to temporal resolution*
  Temporal resolution = frame rate
  High frame rate = shallow depth
  Frame rate depends on the number of scan lines. Therefore while imaging moving structures, make your image as small as possible.
  Short pulse duration = short spatial pulse length [SPL] = better longitudinal [radial] resolution)

Q.162 Highest velocity is seen in
  (a) Proximal to stenosis
  (b) In the center of lumen
  (c) At the wall
  (d) Distal to stenosis

Q.163 What happens to wavelength while using ultrasound harmonics?
  (a) Doubled
  (b) Quadrupled
  (c) Halved
  (d) No change
  (*Hint: THI uses twice the fundamental frequency*)

Q.164 IVC may be pushed anteriorly by
  (a) Spine
  (b) Right renal artery
  (c) Lymph nodes
  (d) Aorta

Q.165 *Shot gun* sign refers to
  (a) Dilated pancreatic duct
  (b) Dilated CBD
  (c) Dilated IHBR
  (d) Dilated portal vein

Q.166 Width of USG beam depends on
  (a) Amplitude
  (b) Depth
  (c) Frequency
  (d) wavelength

Q.167 The benign invasion of endometrium into uterine myometrium
  (a) Leiomyomas
  (b) Endometriosis

(c) Adenomyosis

(d) Asherman's syndrome

Q.168 Minimum lateral resolution of the system is 2.5 millimeters. What is the approximate diameter of a disc-shaped unfocused PZ crystal?

(a) 2.5 millimeters

(b) 5 millimeters

(c) 1 millimeters

(d) 1 centimeter

(*Hint: The beam converges to its narrowest width, which is half the width of the transducer.*

The beam width at the focus is half the diameter of the crystal.)

Q.169 Common benign lesions in cervix

(a) Bartholin's cyst

(b) Gartner's cyst

(c) Nabothian cysts

(d) All of the above

Q.170 Patient with PID has increased risk of

(a) Ectopic pregnancy

(b) H. mole

(c) Patau's syndrome

(d) Endometriosis

Q.171 How many lobes of liver are there as per Couinaud

(a) 2

(b) 3

(c) 6

(d) 8

Q.172 Shape of a sector transducer is

(a) Trapezoidal

(b) Rectangular

(c) Circular

(d) Any of the above

Q.173 An average propagation velocity of sound in human body is

(a) 1,480 meters per second

(b) 330 meters per second

(c) 1,540 meters per second

(d) 5,000 meters per second

Q.174 Which of the following causes least attenuation of sound beam?

(a) Air

(b) Bone

(c) Soft tissue

(d) Stone

(*Hint: Attenuation is reduction in intensity of sound waves as it passes through the tissues. Occurs due to absorption, scattering, and reflection of sound beam.*

Proportional to insonating frequency. High frequency probe—Rapid attenuation and less penetration

Attenuation value of water—0

Attenuation value of Soft tissue—0.7

Attenuation value of Bone—5

Attenuation value of Air—10)

Q.175 Which of the following has the least intensity output?

(a) Color flow imaging

(b) Gray-scale imaging

(c) Duplex imaging

(d) Color-coded inversion imaging.

Q.176 Cavitation as biological effect in ultrasound implies

(a) Tissue heating

(b) Interaction of sound waves with microscopic gas bubbles in the tissues

(c) Formation of cavity in liver

(d) Formation of cavity in lungs

Q.177 Mechanical index is a measure of

(a) Tissue heating

(b) Cavitation effect

(c) Mechanical stress on transducer

(d) None of the above

Q.178 Good quality image requires

(a) Broad Bandwidth

(b) Short SPL

(c) Low Q factor

(d) All of the above

Q.179 What will be the approximate frequency of sound wave in human soft tissue with a wavelength of 0.3 millimeters?

(a) 5 MHz

(b) 10 MHz

(c) 12 MHz

(d) 15 MHz

(*Hint: frequency = propagation speed/wavelength*

Adjusting the units,

frequency = 1.540/0.3 = 5 MHz)

Q.180 Tissue heating occurs due to

(a) Specular reflection

(b) Diffuse reflection

(c) Absorption

(d) Refraction

Q.181 As an ultrasound pulse passes through a tissue in a patient's body it will undergo change in all except
(a) Amplitude
(b) Intensity
(c) Physical size
(d) Frequency

Q.182 Changing from 10 MHz to 3.5 MHz ultrasound transducer
(a) Deeper penetration
(b) Less penetration
(c) Rapid attenuation
(d) Longer ultrasound pulses

Q.183 High frequency transducer is selected for
(a) Better image detail
(b) Obese person
(c) Deeper penetration
(d) All of the above

Q.184 Increasing the number of lines (scan line density) in the image will
(a) Increase the depth of imaging
(b) Decrease the visibility of anatomical detail
(c) Increase the visibility of anatomical detail
(d) Increase the pulse velocity

Q.185 Artifact produced by fluid filled compartment:
(a) Shadowing
(b) Enhancement
(c) Reverberation
(d) Mirror imaging

Q.186 The lowest rate of ultrasound absorption occurs in
(a) Fat
(b) Stone
(c) Air
(d) Bone

Q.187 While changing an ultrasound gain, echoes at a depth of approximately 5 centimeters appear comparatively weaker. Which control will be used to increase the image brightness?
(a) Focusing
(b) Time-gain compensation
(c) Dynamic range
(d) Beam intensity

Q.188 Intensity of an ultrasound beam is measured in
(a) Rad
(b) Sievert
(c) Watts
(d) Heat units

Q.189 Sonographically, arteries tend to be
(a) Thin walled
(b) Collapsible
(c) Both (a) and (b)
(d) Pulsatile

Q.190 A typical pulse duration in ultrasound is
(a) 0.5 microsecond
(b) 0.5 millisecond
(c) 0.5 second
(d) 5 seconds

Q.191 Most commonly used type of probe for echocardiography
(a) Curved array
(b) Phased array
(c) Linear array
(d) Transvaginal probe

Q.192 If a given probe has a depth of penetration of 20 centimeters when it operates at 5.0 MHz what would you expect the depth of penetration would be, if its frequency was increased to 10 MHz?
(a) 20 centimeters
(b) 40 centimeters
(c) 10 centimeters
(d) 5 centimeters

Q.193 Evaluation of which structure is best with high-frequency transducers:
(a) Abdominal aorta
(b) Common carotid artery
(c) Distal superficial femoral vein
(d) A palpable lump on the dorsal wrist

Q.194 Which transducer is superior for imaging pediatric abdomen?
(a) 7.5 MHz curved array
(b) 2 MHz linear array
(c) 5 MHz curved array
(d) 5 MHz sector

Q.195 Sound can propagate as
(a) Shear waves
(b) Longitudinal waves
(c) Surface waves
(d) All of the above

Q.196 Membranous obstruction of IVC, hyperco-
agulation states, hepatic vein compression all
are suggestive of
(a) Portal hypertension
(b) Kaposi's sarcoma
(c) Budd Chiari syndrome
(d) Cirrhosis

Q.197 Chaperone is
(a) Consent by the patient
(b) Witness for both patient and doctor
(c) Artifacts noted in USG machine
(d) Quality assurance of machine

Q.198 Form F under PCPNDT is for
(a) Nondisclosure of sex of the fetus

(b) Invasive procedures
(c) Registration of USG clinic
(d) All of the above

Q.199 Right hepatic space is also called
(a) Cul-de-sac
(b) Pouch of Douglas
(c) Morrison's pouch
(d) None of the above

Q.200 All are important causes of RLQ pain in
abdomen except
(a) Appendicitis
(b) Ruptured ectopic
(c) Diverticulitis
(d) Abdominal tuberculosis

Answer Key

1.	(b)	37.	(b)
2.	(c)	38.	(c)
3.	(d)	39.	(d)
4.	(d)	40.	(b)
5.	(a)	41.	(b)
6.	(b)	42.	(b)
7.	(a)	43.	(c)
8.	(b)	44.	(a)
9.	(c)	45.	(a)
10.	(a)	46.	(b)
11.	(b)	47.	(c)
12.	(c)	48.	(c)
13.	(d)	49.	(c)
14.	(b)	50.	(b)
15.	(a)	51.	(c)
16.	(c)	52.	(b)
17.	(d)	53.	(b)
18.	(a)	54.	(c)
19.	(d)	55.	(b)
20.	(c)	56.	(b)
21.	(c)	57.	(c)
22.	(a)	58.	(b)
23.	(d)	59.	(b)
24.	(c)	60.	(a)
25.	(a)	61.	(a)
26.	(b)	62.	(c)
27.	(a)	63.	(b)
28.	(b)	64.	(b)
29.	(c)	65.	(a)
30.	(b)	66.	(a)
31.	(b)	67.	(a)
32.	(b)	68.	(b)
33.	(c)	69.	(b)
34.	(d)	70.	(b)
35.	(c)	71.	(c)
36.	(a)	72.	(c)

73.	(a)		124.	(b)
74.	(b)		125.	(d)
75.	(c)		126.	(b)
76.	(d)		127.	(d)
77.	(c)		128.	(b)
78.	(a)		129.	(c)
79.	(d)		130.	(a)
80.	(a)		131.	(b)
81.	(a)		132.	(c)
82.	(a)		133.	(a)
83.	(b)		134.	(b)
84.	(d)		135.	(a)
85.	(a)		136.	(c)
86.	(b)		137.	(b)
87.	(d)		138.	(d)
88.	(c)		139.	(c)
89.	(d)		140.	(d)
90.	(a)		141.	(d)
91.	(b)		142.	(c)
92.	(c)		143.	(a)
93.	(a)		144.	(b)
94.	(d)		145.	(c)
95.	(a)		146.	(d)
96.	(d)		147.	(a)
97.	(b)		148.	(c)
98.	(c)		149.	(a)
99.	(b)		150.	(b)
100.	(c)		151.	(d)
101.	(b)		152.	(a)
102.	(a)		153.	(a)
103.	(d)		154.	(b)
104.	(a)		155.	(c)
105.	(c)		156.	(c)
106.	(b)		157.	(d)
107.	(c)		158.	(a)
108.	(c)		159.	(a)
109.	(d)		160.	(b)
110.	(b)		161.	(d)
111.	(c)		162.	(b)
112.	(a)		163.	(c)
113.	(d)		164.	(c)
114.	(a)		165.	(b)
115.	(b)		166.	(b)
116.	(c)		167.	(c)
117.	(c)		168.	(b)
118.	(a)		169.	(c)
119.	(b)		170.	(a)
120.	(a)		171.	(b)
121.	(c)		172.	(a)
122.	(d)		173.	(c)
123.	(a)		174.	(c)

175.	(b)	188.	(c)
176.	(b)	189.	(d)
177.	(b)	190.	(a)
178.	(d)	191.	(b)
179.	(a)	192.	(c)
180.	(c)	193.	(d)
181.	(d)	194.	(a)
182.	(a)	195.	(d)
183.	(a)	196.	(c)
184.	(b)	197.	(b)
185.	(b)	198.	(a)
186.	(a)	199.	(c)
187.	(b)	200.	(c)

Case Reports

EMERGENCY CASES

Case 1

A 23-year-old female landed up in our department with BP 80/65 complaining of excruciating right lower quadrant (RLQ) pain and vaginal spotting. Her urinary pregnancy test was positive. Sample was sent for biochemical evaluation.

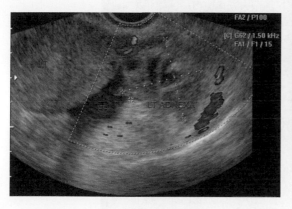

USG reveals:
> Thickened endometrial stripe in an otherwise empty uterine cavity.
> Heterogeneous lesion in left adnexa. Right ovary appears normal.
> Free fluid in Morrison's pouch and in pelvic cavity.

Findings were s/o ruptured ectopic pregnancy.

Aggressive resuscitation with immediate operative management was done.

Case 2

A 40-year-old male patient with history of road traffic accident. His BP is 90/65 and heart rate is 130 beats per minute and is complaining of severe pain in abdomen.

FAST scan was done as per protocol for trauma evaluation.

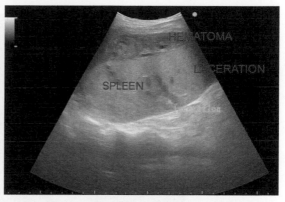

USG abdomen reveals:
> Mild amount of free fluid in perihepatic space
> Multiple linear hypoechoic areas mainly involving the mid and upper pole of spleen
> Heterogeneous collection of approximate 2 centimeters depth in the splenic subcapsular region
> Involving less than 50% of surface

Multiple lacerations with subcapsular hematoma and no active extravasation of contrast (suggesting no active bleed) was further confirmed by contrast enhanced computed tomography (CECT) of abdomen. Hence, patient was managed conservatively.

Discussion

Grading of the splenic trauma by American Association for the Surgery of Trauma (AAST).

- *Grade I*
  Subcapsular hematoma <10% of surface area
  Laceration <1 centimeter depth
- *Grade II*
  Subcapsular hematoma 10%–50% of surface area
  Intraparenchymal hematoma <5 centimeters in diameter
  Laceration 1–3 centimeters depth
- *Grade III*
  Subcapsular hematoma >50% of surface area or expanding
  Intraparenchymal hematoma >5 centimeters or expanding
  Laceration >3 centimeters depth
  Ruptured subcapsular or parenchymal hematoma
- *Grade IV*
  Laceration involving segmental or hilar vessels with major devascularization (>25% of spleen)
- *Grade V*
  Shattered spleen
  Hilar vascular injury with splenic devascularization

Case 3

A 33-year-old male patient came to the emergency room with complaints of severe dysuria and irritative voiding symptoms since early morning.

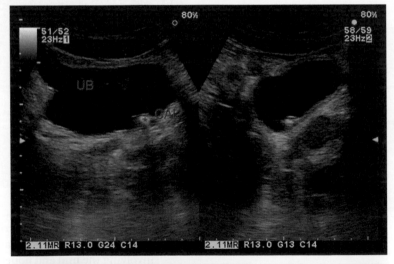

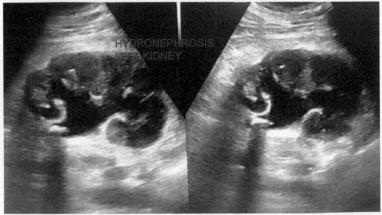

USG findings: Left-sided pelvicalyceal system and ureter appeared to be mildly dilated with an echogenic focus of size 1.2 centimeters, casting posterior acoustic shadow was seen at left vesicoureteric junction. The echogenic foci showed twinkling artifact on color Doppler.

Findings s/o left-sided vesico–ureteric junction (VUJ) calculus with left-sided mild hydroureteronephrosis.

Symptomatic treatment with IV fluids and pain control was provided immediately. Sent to urology department for follow-up since renal function tests (RFTs) were normal and no signs of infection were present.

Discussion

Renal colic refers to a pattern of abdominal pain usually caused by ureteric calculi. While the term really only directly applies to pain symptomatology, it is often used synonymously by patients and health professionals alike to imply the specific pathology of ureteric calculus, despite the fact that there are other potential causes for renal colic (e.g., blood clots, sloughed papilla, sickle cell disease).

Ureteric calculi or stones are those lying within the ureter at any point from the pelvi-ureteric junction (PUJ) to the VUJ.

Patients with ureteric calculus may present with peristaltic pain (renal colic), hematuria, nausea, and vomiting.

The quality and location of pain are dependent on the calculi's location within the ureter.

- Calculi at PUJ may cause deep flank pain without radiation to the groin due to distension of the renal capsule.
- Upper ureteral calculi—Pain radiates to the flank and lumbar areas.
- Midureteric calculi—Pain radiates anteriorly.
- Distal ureteric calculi—Pain radiates to the groin via referred pain from the genitofemoral or ilioinguinal nerves.
- VUJ calculi—Irritative voiding symptoms such as dysuria and urinary frequency.

Up to 80% of renal calculi are formed by calcium stones. Other types include struvite, uric acid and cysteine, and mucoprotein (matrix), xanthine or indinavir stones (rarely) may be encountered.

Calculi forms when stone-forming substances such as calcium or uric acid supersaturates the urine, initiating crystal formation or when such substances deposit on the renal medullary interstitium forming a Randall's plaque, which erodes into the papillary urothelium forming a calculus.

Risk factors include the following: history of prior ureteric calculi and family history, low fluid intake, frequent urinary tract infections, and medications that may crystallize the urine.

Case 4

A 43-year-old female patient came with chief complaints of severe abdominal pain since 1 day. There is history of nonpassage of stools and flatus since 3 days associated with recurrent vomiting.

On examination, the abdomen was distended with rebound tenderness.

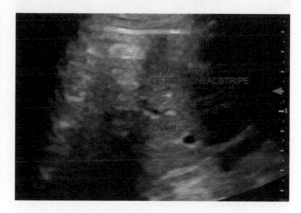

USG findings: There is evidence of enhancement of peritoneal stripe on the anterior surface of liver. There is mild amount of hypoechoic free fluid with internal echoes and few air foci also noted in the peritoneal cavity. Findings are s/o hollow viscus perforation.

An erect chest X-ray PA view was done, which demonstrated free gas under the right hemidiaphragm, consistent with the findings seen on ultrasound.

Discussion

Pneumoperitoneum (gas within the peritoneal cavity) often signifies critical illness with multiple causes and numerous mimics; the most common cause being the disruption of the wall of a hollow viscus. The other causes include peptic ulcer disease, ischemic bowel, appendicitis, diverticulitis, mechanical perforation, trauma, iatrogenic, and postoperative free intraperitoneal gas.

Case 5

A 34-year-old male patient came with symptoms of colicky abdominal pain, abdominal distension, recurrent vomiting, and nonpassage of stools and flatus since 2 days.

X-ray abdomen erect of the patient was done. It showed multiple air fluid levels within the small bowel loops.

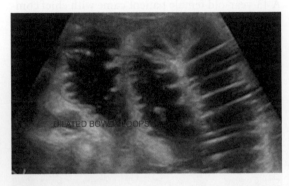

USG findings: Few dilated jejunal loops with contents showing to and fro motion. A distal collapsed segment was seen in proximal ileum, proximal to which bowel appears dilated.
Findings are s/o small bowel (Jejunal) obstruction.

Discussion

Intestinal obstructions are common and are usually divided as per the site of obstruction. Imaging appearances and treatment depends on the underlying pathology.

Causes of bowel obstruction:

- Adhesions from previous abdominal surgery (most common cause)
- Hernias containing bowel
- Inflammatory bowel disease causing adhesions or strictures
- Neoplasms, benign, or malignant
- Intussusception in children
- Volvulus
- Superior mesenteric artery syndrome, compression of the duodenum by the superior mesenteric artery, and the abdominal aorta

- Ischemic strictures
- Foreign bodies (e.g., gallstones in gallstone ileus, swallowed objects)
- Intestinal atresia
- Diverticulitis/Diverticulosis
- Constipation
- Fecal impaction
- Intestinal pseudo-obstruction

Case 6

A 35-year-old female patient presented with acute onset of severe pain in the epigastric region since 2 days associated with history of vomiting. The pain was radiating to the back. There is history of fever since 1 day. Her serum amylase levels were 780 mIU/mL.

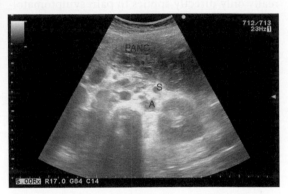

On USG: Pancreas appear bulky in size and heterogeneously hypoechoic in echotexture with few cystic/necrotic areas. Few small pockets of hypoechoic fluid collection in the peripancreatic region.
Findings are s/o acute pancreatitis.
Patient was managed conservatively and kept on follow-up.

Case 7

A 17-year-old male presented with acute onset pain in the right iliac fossa region with fever and vomiting since 1 day. Blood reports showed leukocytosis.

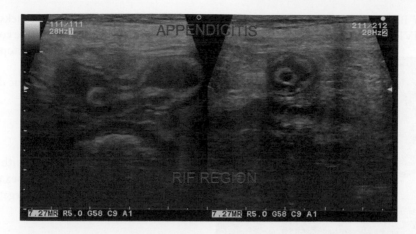

On USG: There is a tubular, blind-ended, nonperistaltic, and noncompressible structure measuring 11 millimeters in diameter arising from the base of cecum with inflamed surrounding mesentery.

Findings are s/o acute appendicitis.

Patient was managed conservatively and referred to the surgery department for further evaluation and operative management.

Case 8

A 40-year-old fatty female presented with pain in the right upper abdomen.

USG reveals a large gallstone with mildly thickened gallbladder wall and contracted lumen.

Findings are s/o acute biliary colic due to cholelithiasis with acute cholecystitis.

Patient was managed symptomatically and referred to the surgery department for planned evaluation.

Case 9

A 54-year-old male patient complains of breathlessness, chest pain, and dizziness since few days but aggravates suddenly to land him in our emergency department. No history of trauma was

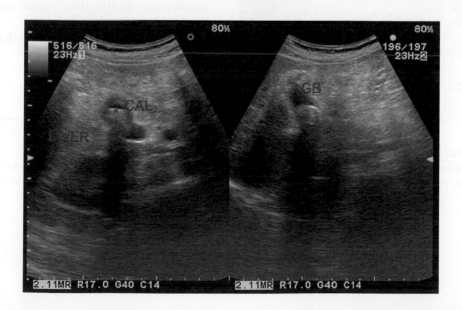

reported. His BP was 90/65, heart sounds were muffled, and JVP was raised.

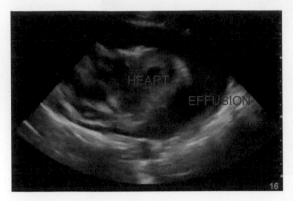

USG reveals large pericardial effusion.
Findings were s/o pericardial effusion with impaired cardiac function s/o cardiac tamponade.
The image-guided drainage of effusion was done and referred to cardiology department for further management.

Case 10

A 24-year-old female patient presented with the history of lower abdominal pain and irregular periods. Her urine pregnancy test was positive.

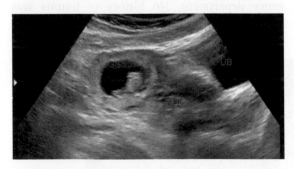

USG: Uterus was mildly bulky with thick endometrium measuring 14 millimeters. Gestational sac with yolk sac and fetal pole of mean sac

diameter corresponding to 6 weeks 3 days with good cardiac activity seen in the cornua.
Findings were suggestive of live ectopic pregnancy.
The patient was referred to obstetric department for emergent evaluation.

Case 11

A 28-year-old female presented with severe lower abdominal pain, nausea, and adnexal tenderness. Her urinary pregnancy test was negative but WBC counts were raised.

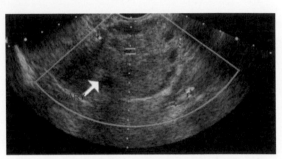

USG reveals
Mildly enlarged hypoechoic right ovary with absence of vascularity.
Mild amount of free fluid in the pelvic cavity.
Findings were s/o ovarian torsion and confirmed on CECT scan, which revealed enlarged, nonenhancing ovary with distended pedicle surrounding fat stranding, edema, and free fluid.
Patient was referred to the gynecology department for operative management.

ROUTINE CASES

Case 12

A young 16-year-old female patient complains of irregular and delayed periods since 3 months.

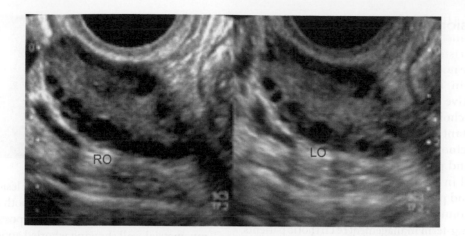

On USG: The transabdominal ultrasound images reveal bilateral mildly bulky ovaries with multiple follicles in each ovary, more than 10 on each side. The echogenicity of stroma appears to be mildly raised. Uterus appears to be normal. Final diagnosis—Polycystic ovarian disease (PCOD).

Discussion

The Stein Leventhal (polycystic ovarian syndrome) syndrome is usually present in obese, hirsute females with history of amenorrhea/irregular periods. Patients require two out of three Rotterdam criteria for diagnosis.

Rotterdam criteria:

1. Ovarian dysfunction (oligoanovulation and or polycystic ovaries).
2. Presence of hyperandrogenism (clinical or biochemical—LH/FSH).
3. Follicle count on imaging.

The typical sonographic appearance includes bilaterally enlarged ovaries (2–3 times bulkier than normal, but up to 30% may have normal-sized ovaries) with multiple peripherally arranged small follicles of size 0.5–0.8 meters (String of pearls/Necklace sign) and an increased stromal echogenicity.

Case 13

A 55-year-old alcoholic male patient presented with abdominal distension since 2 months and yellowish discoloration of eyes since 1 month.

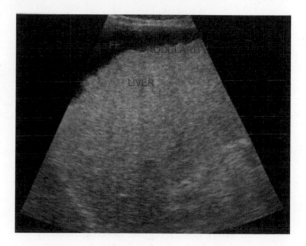

On USG:
  Liver is shrunken in size with coarse echotexture, surface irregularity, and nodularity.
  Edematous gallbladder.
  Moderate ascites.
  Portal vein is normal in caliber.
Final diagnosis—Chronic liver disease.

Discussion

Characteristic findings of liver cirrhosis in ultrasound are nodular liver surface due to hypoechoic nodules in liver parenchyma, which represent regenerative nodules of cirrhotic liver. Detection of hypoechoic nodule more than 10 millimeters is important in the early diagnosis of hepatocellular carcinoma. USG detection of splenomegaly, ascites, and portosystemic collaterals is easy and beneficial in the management of esophagogastric varices and portosystemic encephalopathy.

Ultrasound is useful in the noninvasive diagnosis and long-term management of cirrhotic patients.

Case 14

A 55-year-old female patient came with complaints of hard painless lump in the left breast since 2 months. The lump had increased in size in the last 15 days.

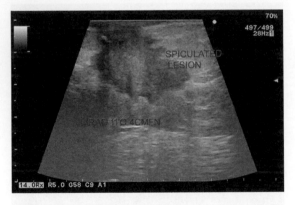

On USG: There is an irregular heterogeneously hypoechoic lesion with spiculated margins seen in upper inner quadrant of left breast extending from 10 to 11 o'clock position. The lesion showed microcalcifications and internal vascularity within it.

Findings were suggestive of carcinoma breast. Patient was advised FNA biopsy for further evaluation.

Case 15

A 35-year-old female came with chief complaints of lump in the abdomen since 5 months. There was associated menorrhagia and pain. There was no history of weight loss.

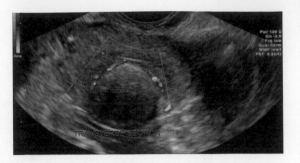

On USG: A well-defined heteroechoic lesion of size 7.9 × 7.2 centimeters with smooth and regular wall seen arising from the posterior myometrial wall showing whorled appearance. Bilateral adnexa appear to be normal in size, shape, and echotexture. Findings were s/o uterine fibroid.

Discussion

Uterine leiomyomas (fibroids) are benign tumors of myometrial origin and are the most common solid benign uterine neoplasm.

Often asymptomatic and discovered incidentally, they rarely cause a diagnostic quandary. Signs and symptoms associated with fibroids include abnormal vaginal bleeding, pain, infertility, or palpable masses.

Fibroids may have a number of locations within or external to the uterus.

LEIOMYOMA CLASSIFICATION

Intramural	Confined to the myometrium
Submucosal	Projecting into the uterine cavity
Subserosal	Projecting from the peritoneal surface

Subserosal fibroids may be pedunculated and predominantly extrauterine, simulating an adnexal mass. Any fibroid may undergo atrophy, internal hemorrhage, fibrosis, and calcification.

They can also undergo several types of degeneration: *hyaline degeneration* being the most common type. Others include *cystic degeneration, myxoid degeneration, and red/carneous degeneration* (hemorrhagic infarction), which can occur particularly during pregnancy and may present with an acute abdominal pain.

Ultrasound is used to diagnose the presence and monitor the growth of fibroids. Uncomplicated leiomyomas are usually hypoechoic, but can be isoechoic, or even hyperechoic compared to normal myometrium. Calcification is seen as echogenic foci with shadowing. Cystic areas of necrosis or degeneration may be seen.

Case 16

A 10-year-old female presented with intermittent pain in abdomen since 2 months, predominantly in the right lumbar region. She also complained of pruritis and icterus since 3 months. There is history of vomiting since 2 days.

She gave no history of melena or hematemesis and had no gastrointestinal complaints.

Laboratory findings included mild elevation of total and direct serum bilirubin and raised levels of alkaline phosphatase.

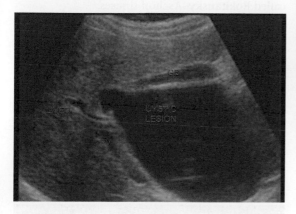

On USG:
   A well-defined cystic lesion measuring approximately 8.4 × 6.3 centimeters seen anterior to portal vein. Common bile duct (CBD) was not visualized separately.
   Mild hepatomegaly.
   Gallbladder is visualized separately.
CECT abdomen reveals cystic dilatation of CBD and intrahepatic biliary radicles along with hepatomegaly. The findings confirmed type IV-A choledochal cyst.

Discussion

Choledochal cysts denote rare congenital cystic dilatations of the biliary tree. Diagnosis depends on the exclusion of other conditions (e.g., tumors, gallstone, inflammation) as a cause of biliary duct dilatation.

Although they can be found at any age, 60% are diagnosed before the age of 10 years with a strong female predilection (M:F ratio of 1:4).

Typical presentation includes the triad of pain, jaundice, and abdominal mass, which is however only present in ~45% of cases

Commonly accepted classification currently by Todani et al. is described in Chapter 4.

Case 17

A 25-year-old female presented with chief complaints of pain in abdomen predominantly in the pelvic region since 2 months, feeling of lump in abdomen since 1½ months. There is history of fever since 3 days.

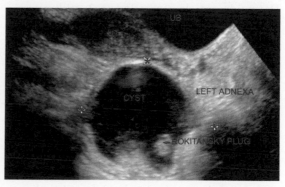

Imaging findings on USG: A well-defined, avascular, cystic lesion of approximate size 5.6 × 5.4 centimeters seen in the left adnexal region with Rokitansky (echogenic) plug within it.

Discussion

Cystic teratomas or dermoids account for 10%–15% of all ovarian tumors and are bilateral in 10% of the cases. They arise from totipotent germ cells and are composed of mature epithelial elements: a combination of skin, hair, sebum, desquamated epithelium, and teeth.

Dermoids are relatively soft masses and may be difficult to palpate, so are frequently either missed or underestimated in size. If large, a dermoid may torse, and then present as an acute abdominal pain. They are rarely malignant.

Dermoids vary in size and echogenicity. Depending on the extent and admixture of their epithelial elements, the ultrasound patterns can vary markedly, even within a single mass. There are however some typical patterns. The two *classic* dermoid appearances are the *tip of the iceberg* sign caused by the absorption of most of the ultrasound beam at the top of the mass (because of multiple internal interfaces) and *dermoid plug* sign, which has the appearance of one or more hyperechoic areas within a hypoechoic mass.

Presence of interlacing linear and punctuate echoes corresponding to crossing strands of hair within the mass is more specific though less frequent.

Rarely, a lipid-fluid level can be identified within the mass and the fluid level may shift position when the patient moves.

Treatment

Dermoids are slow growing (1–2 millimeters a year) and, therefore, some advocate nonsurgical management. Larger lesions are often surgically removed. Many recommend annual follow-up for lesions <7 centimeters to monitor growth, beyond which a resection is advised.

Case 18

A 40-year-old female came with the complaint of intermittent abdominal pain mostly after eating since 1 month, not associated with fever, jaundice, or vomiting. She has no h/o chronic illness such as diabetes, hypertension, tuberculosis, asthma, and so on.

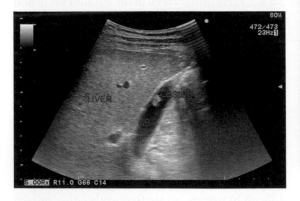

On USG: Small nonmobile outgrowth of the gallbladder mucosal wall toward the lumen without acoustic shadowing is noted. On color Doppler, feeder blood vessel is pathognomic of polyp.

Most polyps are asymptomatic and found incidentally. Most small polyps (less than 1 centimeters) are not premalignant and may remain unchanged for years. However, when small polyps occur with premalignant conditions, such as primary sclerosing cholangitis, they are less likely to be benign. Larger polyps are more likely to turn into adenocarcinomas.

Cholesterolosis represents an outgrowth of the mucosal lining of the gallbladder into finger-like projections due to the excessive accumulation of cholesterol and triglycerides within macrophages in the epithelial lining. These cholesterol polyps account for most benign gallbladder polyp.

Adenomyomatosis represents excessively thick gallbladder wall due to proliferation of subsurface cellular layer. It is characterized by deep folds into the muscularis propria. USG may reveal the thickened gallbladder wall with intramural diverticulae called Rokitansky–Aschoff sinuses.

Case 19

A 60-year-old male patient presented with right upper quadrant pain and abdominal discomfort since 5 months. He also has on and off fever, decreased appetite, and jaundice since 1 month.

Physical examination

On palpation: Liver appears to be enlarged. Yellowish discoloration of sclera and palm.

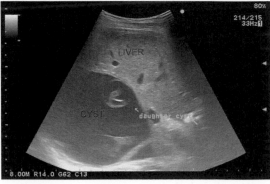

USG findings: A large well-defined cystic lesion is seen in the right lobe of liver and a small cystic lesion (daughter cyst) seen within the lesion. Color Doppler study did not reveal any vascularity within the lesion.

Discussion

Echinococcus granulosus is the most common cause of hydatid disease. It can result in the cyst formation anywhere in the body. Liver is the most common site followed by lungs.

Sonographic findings in hepatic hydatid disease (WHO 2001 classification):

- *CL*: Unilocular anechoic cystic lesion without any internal echoes and septations
- *CE 1*: Uniformly anechoic cyst with fine echoes settled in it (*Hydatid sand*)
- *CE 2* (*Active stage*): Cyst with multiple septations (Rosette/Honeycomb appearance)
- *CE 3* (*Transitional stage*): Unilocular cyst with daughter cysts with detached laminated membranes (Water lily sign)
- *CE 4* (*Degenerative stage*): Mixed hypo- and hyperechoic contents with absence of daughter cysts (Ball of wool sign)
- *CE 5* (*Inactive and infertile stage*): Curved, thick, partially, or completely calcified wall

Case 20

Clinical presentation: A 45-year-old female patient with history of altered bowel habits and bleeding per rectum since 1 month.

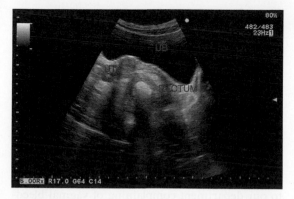

On USG: Circumferential thickening of rectum with obliteration of its lumen and proximal dilation of sigmoid colon. She was further evaluated by colonoscopy and adenocarcinoma was confirmed on histopathology.

Case 21

A 30-year-old male presented with chief complaints of right upper quadrant pain since 2 months, high fever, malaise, and weakness.

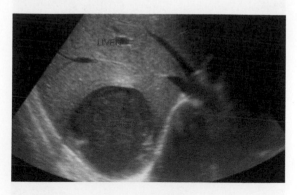

On USG: Hypoechoic, avascular, rounded lesion of volume approximately 290 cubic centimeters seen in the right lobe of liver with well-defined walls and low-level internal echoes. The wall appears to be thin and regular. There is mild hepatomegaly. Rest of the liver parenchyma appears to be normal in echotexture.

USG-guided aspiration of the lesion was done, which showed anchovy sauce pus. On histopathological examination (HPE), the contents were confirmed to be amoebic in nature.

Discussion

Hepatic abscesses are focal collections of necrotic inflammatory tissue caused by bacterial, parasitic, or fungal pathogens.

An amoebic hepatic abscess is caused by *Entamoeba histolytica*.

Patients may feel general malaise or present with frank sepsis and right upper quadrant pain.

CT: Usually appear as rounded, well-defined, hypodense lesions with an enhancing rim, and a peripheral zone of edema with the wall thickness around 4–16 millimeters. The central abscess cavity can show septations and/or fluid–debris levels.

Gas within an abscess suggests complications such as hepatobronchial or hepatocolic fistula.

Drainage may be required, preponderantly in larger abscesses, which are at risk of spontaneous rupture into the peritoneal, pleural, or pericardial spaces.

Case 22

Routine ultrasound of a 55-year-old male patient, a known case of lung carcinoma, was done.

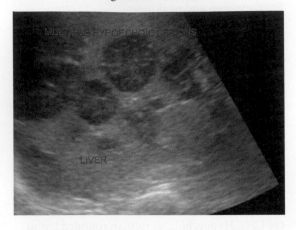

On USG: Multiple, well-defined, avascular, rounded, hypoechoic lesions noted in the liver. The rest of the liver parenchyma appeared normal in echotexture.

On biopsy, the lesion proved to be metastatic deposits from adenocarcinoma.

For detail refer Chapter 2.

Case 23

A 23-year-old female patient presented with history of painless lump in her left breast since 5 months. There was no history of any increase in the size of the lump.

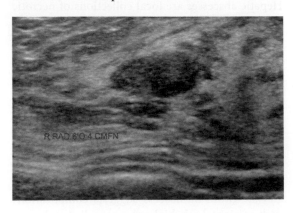

On USG: A well–defined, homogenously hypoechoic lesion of approximate size 32 × 19 millimeters seen in the right upper quadrant at 10 o'clock position. The lesion showed peripheral vascularity. No evidence of any enlarged intramammary and axillary lymph nodes. Rest of the breast parenchyma and contralateral breast appeared normal.

Impression: Findings are suggestive of fibroadenoma.

Case 24

A young girl with history of amenorrhea, palpable lower abdominal swelling, and cyclical abdominal pain reported to our department for USG abdomen. Her secondary sexual characters were normal for her age.

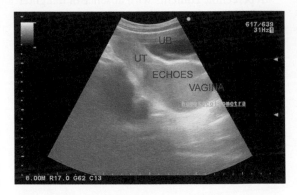

Her USG revealed distended uterus and vagina filled with blood (hematometrocolpos). Findings were suggestive of imperforate hymen. She was sent to gynecology department for further evaluation and surgical management.

Case 25

A middle-aged postmenopausal female presented to our department complaining of vaginal bleeding. She was obese and diabetic.

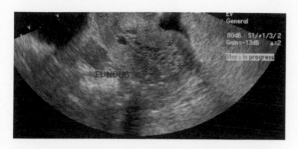

Her USG (TVS) revealed thickened heterogeneous endometrium. Bilateral ovaries appeared normal but atrophic.

Findings were s/o carcinoma endometrium and were confirmed after biopsy.

Discussion

Any postmenopausal female with vaginal bleeding and thickened heterogeneous endometrium should be considered as malignancy until proven otherwise.

All the cases have been discussed in their respective sections.

Findings were s/o carcinoma endometrium and were confirmed after biopsy.

H/e USG (TVS) revealed thickened heterogeneous endometrium. Bilateral ovaries appeared normal but atrophic.

Discussion

Any postmenopausal female with vaginal bleeding and thickened heterogeneous endometrium should be considered as malignancy until proven otherwise.

All the cases have been discussed in their respective sections.

Glossary

A mode: amplitude mode

acoustic enhancement: structures that attenuate USG beam less than the surrounding tissues lead to too bright echoes behind them. Usually seen in cystic lesions

acoustic shadowing: reduction in intensity of ultrasound (black zone) deep to a strong reflector (such as gas or foreign body) or extensive absorption in bones

anechoic: completely black without any echoes

axial resolution: ability to separate structures *one over the other along (parallel)* the axis of USG beam

azimuth/elevation resolution: determined by the slice thickness in the plane perpendicular to both beam and to transducer

B mode: brightness mode (gray scale, real time)

chaperone: a person who acts as a witness for both a patient and a medical practitioner during a medical examination or procedure

continuous wave (CW) Doppler: sound wave is continuously transmitted from one piezoelectric crystal and received by a separate transducer

contrast resolution: depicted by different shades of gray in the image

curie temperature: the temperature above which crystal loses its PE properties/polarization

Doppler shift: change in frequency of signals when there is relative motion between the source and the reflector

duty factor: time spent sending signals/time spent receiving signals

echogenicity: depends on density of structure, number, and type of reflectors within it and its interaction with sound beam

echotexture: depicted by different shades of gray

elastography: when a mechanical compression/vibration is applied, the tumor deforms less than the surrounding tissue, that is, the strain in tumor is less

focused assessment with sonography for trauma (FAST): a focused, goal-directed sonography examination of abdomen

frequency: the number of cycles per second; measured in Hz (Hertz)

high-intensity focused ultrasound (HIFU): absorption of ultrasound energy in the tissue during transmission induces cavitation damage and coagulative thermal necrosis

homogeneous echotexture: similar shades of gray

hyperechoic: white with high-level echoes

hypoechoic: low-level echoes, less gray than the surrounding parenchyma

inhomogenous/heterogenous echotexture: different shades of gray in a tissue

isoechoic: mid-level echoes, similar to surrounding parenchyma

lateral resolution: ability to separate structures *side by side at the same depth*; in the plane *perpendicular* to beam axis and parallel to the transducer

longitudinal waves: ultrasound waves with a motion parallel to the direction of wave propagation in a medium

M mode: motion mode

piezoelectric crystal: main component of a transducer (located near the transducer's face). Have the unique ability to respond to the action of an electric field by changing shape (strain)

pulse repetition frequency (PRF): number of transmitted pulses per second

pulse wave (PW) Doppler: sound wave is alternately transmitted and received using only one crystal

pulse-echo principle: pulses of high-frequency sound waves are transmitted to the patient. Echoes returning from various tissue boundaries are detected. The received echo produces an ultrasound image

real-time ultrasound: real-time imaging systems are those that have frame rates fast enough to allow movement to be followed

receiver: receives reflected echoes. Weak pressure changes are converted to electric signals for processing

sample volume (SV): box positioned in the centre of the vessel lumen

spatial resolution: determines the quality of USG image and the ability to differentiate two closely spaced objects as distinct structures

speckle: an intrinsic artifact in an USG image that obscures the underlying anatomy and degrades the spatial and contrast resolution

spectral broadening: chaotic movement of blood cells leading to flow disturbances and multiple velocities filling up the spectral window

temporal resolution: for a moving structure like in obstetric and echocardiography. Also known as frame rate

time-gain compensation (TGC): one of the most important control in the ultrasound unit. In order to compensate for signal loss from the far field, adjustment of sensitivity at each depth is required. This is possible with TGC leading to uniform brightness at all depths for any solid organ, for example, liver

tissue harmonic imaging: higher harmonic frequencies generated by nonlinear wave propagation of USG beam through tissues are used to produce the sonogram. Second harmonic or twice the fundamental frequency is used for imaging

tomographic ultrasound imaging (TUI): displays multiple parallel slices within a volume of dataset; similar to CT and MRI

transmitter: converts electric energy to acoustic pulse, which is transmitted to the patient

ultrasound gel: fluid medium that provides a link between transducer and patient's surface. Coupling agent that transmits USG waves to and from the transducer by eliminating the air b/w the transducer and skin surface

USG transducer: device that converts electrical energy to mechanical energy and vice versa

wall filter: device to suppress very slow flow near the baseline

wavelength: distance between two consecutive waves. Inversely proportion to frequency

Index

Printed and bound by CPI Group (UK) Ltd, Croydon, CR0 4YY
24/10/2024
01778292-0006